PSYCHOTHERAPY
in CLINICAL PRACTICE

Cognitive Behavioral Therapy for Clinicians

PSYCHOTHERAPY
in CLINICAL PRACTICE

Cognitive Behavioral Therapy for Clinicians

DONNA M. SUDAK, M.D.

Associate Professor
Director of Psychotherapy Training
Department of Psychiatry
Drexel University College of Medicine
Philadelphia, Pennsylvania

Supervisor
The Beck Institute for Cognitive Therapy
and Research
Bala Cynwyd, Pennsylvania

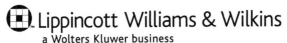 Lippincott Williams & Wilkins
a Wolters Kluwer business
Philadelphia · Baltimore · New York · London
Buenos Aires · Hong Kong · Sydney · Tokyo

Executive Editor: Charles W. Mitchell
Senior Managing Editor: Lisa R. Kairis
Associate Director of Marketing: Adam Glazer
Project Manager: Nicole Walz
Senior Manufacturing Manager: Ben Rivera
Creative Director: Doug Smock
Cover Designer: Lou Fuiano
Production Services: Schawk, Inc.
Printer: RR Donnelley—Crawfordsville

Library of Congress Cataloging-in-Publication Data

Sudak, Donna M.
Cognitive behavioral therapy for clinicians / Donna M. Sudak.
p. ; cm. — (Psychotherapy in clinical practice)
Includes bibliographical references and index.
ISBN 0-7817-6044-5 (alk. paper)
1. Cognitive therapy. 2. Behavior therapy. I. Title. II. Series.
[DNLM: 1. Cognitive Therapy—methods. 2. Mental Disorders—therapy. WM 425.5.C6 S943c 2006]
RC489.C63S83 2006
616.89'142—dc22

2005032554

ISBN 0-7817-6044-5

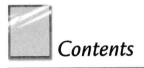

Contents

To my husband, Howard,
the love of my life,
and our daughter, Laura,
who lights each of our days

Introduction

The cognitive behavioral therapies are relatively short-term, goal-directed, problem-focused treatments that are fundamentally based on the model that changing cognitions is possible and leads to behavioral change (Dobson, 2002). The purpose of this monograph is to provide a concise overview of the techniques and conceptual framework of cognitive behavioral therapy, as proposed, researched, and refined by Aaron T. Beck, M.D. It is based on the cognitive model of psychopathology and an individual case conceptualization. The text is designed to be clinically oriented and, whenever possible, case illustrations are used to depict clinical uses of the theoretical material. This is not original material; it is designed to give a beginning practitioner an overview of a well-documented and effective treatment for many psychiatric disorders. Although a rich empirical literature exists that supports the efficacy and effectiveness of these therapeutic interventions, this literature is highlighted and not described in the text. The manual is designed to facilitate beginning clinicians' work with patients using cognitive therapy rather than to provide the evidence supporting the use of the treatment. An important part of the volume is a focus on case conceptualization, as an effort to avoid the use of cognitive techniques without understanding the framework and understanding of the patient must exist to provide truly comprehensive care. What distinguishes therapists as practitioners with different orientations is the way that they conceptualize the development of particular disorders and the formulation that they make of a particular patient and how he or she developed a particular set of problems.

The psychotherapeutic techniques of cognitive therapy are principle-driven, that is, based on the principle that changing cognitions and/or behavior improves symptoms and can help patients with a variety of emotional disorders. Cognitive therapists work to help patients understand that the meanings they attach to their experience derive from their own idiosyncratic perception and that evaluating this meaning for accuracy is frequently a valuable therapeutic tool.

The patients described in the text are fictitious and are designed to reflect the complexity of the patients seen by psychiatry residents. The text uses the terms cognitive therapy and cognitive behavioral therapy interchangeably to refer to cognitive therapy as described by Aaron T. Beck, cognitive therapy being one of the cognitive behavioral therapies.

This text was based on series of lectures developed for the adult psychiatry residents at the Drexel University College of Medicine. Their desire to learn and take good care of patients is a continual inspiration. I owe a great deal to the bravery and patience of my patients, who teach and inspire me to try harder. The book synthesizes my working knowledge of cognitive therapy and is a testimony to the good fortune that I have had in working with and learning from extraordinary teachers, mentors, and colleagues. In particular, I am grateful for my early training at the University of Washington and to my colleagues, including the late Neil Jacobson, Marsha Linehan, Kelly Koerner, and particularly Joan Romano, who gave many helpful suggestions about the manuscript. In Philadelphia, I have had the privilege of being an extramural fellow at The Beck Institute and thank Christine Reilly, Andrew Butler, Leslie Sokol, and the entire staff for creating such an engaging learning environment. I am indebted to the Academy of Cognitive Therapy for their educational support, and in particular, for the chance to learn from Robert Leahy and Jesse Wright. Most invaluable to me as a clinician and teacher has been the chance to work with Judith Beck, whose clear thinking and wonderful teaching set her apart. Finally, I continue to be inspired and grateful to Tim Beck, whose intellect, curiosity, humor, and good sense has changed my life and the lives of many others.

Donna Sudak

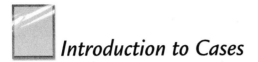

Introduction to Cases

Presented here are the stories of Mr. White, Ms. Green, and Ms. Gray. While fictional, they represent typical patients with commonly seen problems. They will be cited in boxes throughout the text.

CASES

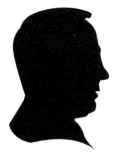

MR. WHITE

Mr. White is a 45-year-old graduate student in economics. He returned to school full-time after working in middle management for several years after college. He presents with symptoms of lifelong dysphoria, low energy, and low self-esteem. The precipitant for his seeking treatment is breaking up with his girlfriend of 9 months. This relationship is his second long-term relationship with a woman. Mr. White was engaged in college. His fiancée broke the engagement just before graduation. Since that breakup, which Mr. White has never felt he understood, Mr. White has dated little, preferring group activities to dating. He met his last girlfriend when he was at the university computer center. She was a sophomore student in the fine arts program. They dated briefly and she went on a summer study abroad; following her return they had an intense and exclusive relationship. At the end of the school year, Mr. White's girlfriend told him she felt the relationship had no future and that she did not want to see him anymore. Mr. White was baffled and distressed by this; they never quarreled, and he describes behaving in a loving way and accommodating her needs throughout the relationship. The only conflict he felt that was significant was that she would accuse him of "keeping his emotional distance."

Since the breakup 5 months ago, Mr. White has been more dysphoric, has had no contact with women, and has avoided some of his old friends. He has been more involved with his studies and has watched TV during much of his free time. He routinely turns down invitations to be with friends or to participate in social gatherings. He has had some increase in his regular weekend marijuana use and is now using it 3 or 4 nights per week. He feels it "takes the edge off."

Mr. White is one of six children, is much younger than his siblings, and is the only boy. His three elder sisters were out of the house throughout most of his childhood; the two sisters closest in age were popular and social. His father was aloof and away on business much of the time, and Mr. White was frequently alone or with his mother, who was volatile and critical of most of what her family members did. Despite her criticism, she would occasionally tell Mr. White that he was the only person she could count on to care for her. This would make her criticism even more hurtful to him. Mr. White never felt

1

confident in school; he was "always hearing about (his siblings') success stories" and felt he never measured up. Additionally, Mr. White had a fairly distinctive port wine birthmark on his neck and was smaller in stature than most of his peers, which he said added to his sense of inferiority. He remembers feeling "devastated" by teasing in fifth or sixth grade and retreating further into his own thoughts. He describes himself as a "chronic underachiever" in school, losing interest in things he starts, but after college he got a fairly good job as an administrator in a software company. He routinely missed opportunities for promotion because he refused, in his words, "to play the game," and declined invitations to meetings, parties, and company events. He made the decision to return to graduate school 2 years ago, and has done reasonably well, although is uncertain what he will do with his degree.

Mr. White made the decision to seek treatment for the first time after this breakup because he felt lonely and unable to move forward in pursuing another relationship. His closest sister, 5 years his senior, also suggested he seek counseling. He feels there is "something missing" and that other people generally seem to be far more capable than he is in social settings.

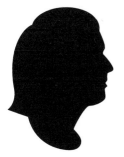

MS. GREEN

Ms. Green is a 43-year-old married woman with three daughters, ages 23, 21, and 16. She has a lifelong history of anxiety and has sought multiple treatments for it from her general practitioner. She changes doctors frequently, feeling like she is not well understood by any of her primary care providers. She has had difficulties with overuse of pain medications and occasionally "borrows" alprazolam from her sister, who also has a history of anxiety. She became more acutely anxious when she found out her eldest daughter was pregnant with her first child. Eight weeks ago, she began to have her first panic attacks, with chest pain, shortness of breath, a sense of impending doom, dizziness, and numbness and tingling in her fingers. She has avoided taking public transportation as a result, despite the fact that she has never had a panic attack on the bus or train. She feels she could "lose control and not get help" were she to have an attack in public. This has meant she has been virtually homebound unless one of her children or her husband accompanies her after they are finished with school or work.

Ms. Green spends much of her day worrying about her family, and her eldest daughter and her pregnancy are a significant focus for her concern. Ms. Green has a lifelong history of abandoning projects because of being worried that bad outcomes will occur; for instance, she quit after the second semester of college when she got concerned that she would never measure up to her fellow students. When told to "relax" by her family, she says that worry is "what good mothers do." She also tends to worry more when she is angry or upset with someone and finds it helps her feel more in control.

Ms. Green is the eldest of six children. Her parents had a volatile relationship; her mother was fairly submissive and her father, who was a security guard, was prone to unpredictable angry outbursts. Finances were always a problem, and her mother took a series of factory jobs to help to supplement the family income, beginning when Ms. Green was 7. Ms. Green was given a significant amount of responsibility for the care of her younger siblings when she was a child and often felt overwhelmed and frightened that "something would go wrong and it would be her fault." Ms. Green was sexually molested at age 10 by a neighbor during a family party and has never told anyone about this incident. She has always thought that there must have been something that she did that caused this to happen. Throughout her adolescence she remained fearful of the possibility that her neighbor would molest her again and avoided social contact during family events. She believes "perfection is possible if you just try harder," and views any emotional difficulties as "weak." She has spent her lifetime caring for her family, but currently feels unable to function effectively and entirely dependent on them for help.

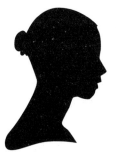

MS. GRAY

Ms. Gray is a 26-year-old art student who has a lengthy history of psychiatric treatment, starting in her middle teens. She is the second of two children and has an older brother who is currently incarcerated for drug-related crimes. Ms. Gray's mother left her father, taking both children with her, when Ms. Gray was 8 years old, and Ms. Gray had little contact with him thereafter. Her mother left her father because of his relentless criticism and cruelty. Ms. Gray witnessed her father hitting her mother on multiple occasions, but she denies being physically abused herself. Her father routinely belittled her and her mother, calling them stupid and worthless. He would laugh at Ms. Gray for crying and told her to "toughen up or shut up." He would often trip her mother or knock books or dishes from Ms. Gray's hands. Ms. Gray was an anxious child, often refusing to go to school. In her middle and high school years she was frequently truant. She was referred for psychotherapy in ninth grade by the school psychologist because of her lack of school attendance and because she had always been an underachiever. She does not recall this therapy as helpful, but says it was "nice to have a grownup to talk to" when her mother was preoccupied with work and her brother's drug problem. Ms. Gray only had therapy until the end of the school year. Ms. Gray started to cut herself with a box cutter at age 16 after a fight with her boyfriend and continues cut herself when she is upset. She made her first suicide attempt at age 17 by overdosing on dexadrine that had been prescribed for her brother for ADHD. She has since made 23 suicide attempts by drug overdose, two of which resulted in intensive care stays. Ms. Gray has generally attempted suicide after stressors like breaking up with boyfriends, fighting with roommates, or during her therapist's vacations.

Ms. Gray has been given a number of psychiatric diagnoses, most recently bipolar disorder and borderline personality disorder. She has taken a variety of psychotropic medications that have done little to alter her mood states, although she says that valproic acid has been somewhat helpful. She has had multiple brief forays into psychiatric treatment, but always drops out. She has never abused drugs, but binge drinks when she is upset. Her mother has supported her financially, and she is currently enrolled on a scholarship in a prestigious art school. The current crisis that brings her to treatment is that her father, who has cancer and is dying, has recently contacted her. He wants her to come live with him and take care of him, and he has told her that she "owes him that much." Following his phone call, Ms. Gray took an overdose of 20 diphenhydramine with no subsequent medical treatment. She was referred to her current therapist by her previous therapist, who refuses to see her again, and who has told her that she has no more ideas about how to help her.

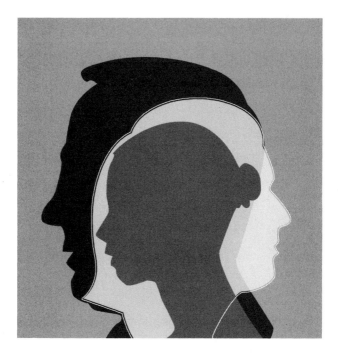

Foundations of Cognitive Therapy

Historical Development of Cognitive Therapy

Aaron T. Beck and Albert Ellis described the core concepts of cognitive behavioral therapy (CBT) in the 1960s. With more than 300 controlled trials supporting its efficacy, cognitive therapy, as defined by Judith Beck (Butler & Beck, 2000), is the psychotherapeutic treatment that has the most empirical support. Although the original treatment was developed for depression, the practical problem-solving orientation and usefulness of CBT led many researchers to adapt it from the original framework and use it for other psychiatric conditions, including hypochondriasis, bulimia nervosa and panic disorder, social phobia, and generalized anxiety disorder. Dialectical behavior therapy, a form of cognitive behavior therapy, has robust empirical support in treating significant symptoms of borderline personality disorder. Schizophrenia and bipolar disorder have significantly improved outcomes when adjunctive cognitive therapy is added to standard pharmacotherapy. CBT has also been tested and found to be effective as a treatment in obsessive–compulsive disorder, posttraumatic stress disorder, and simple phobia; the emphasis in the cognitive behavioral treatment of these disorders is somewhat more behavioral, with an understanding of the perpetuating disturbances in the patient's thinking. Many therapists use the CBT framework of identifying and questioning maladaptive and invalid perceptions and modifying the accompanying behavioral disturbance. As defined by Beck, the therapeutic framework requires the therapist to conceptualize individual patients based on particular developmental experiences, as well by incorporating the genetic and biological underpinnings of disturbances. Cognitive therapy emphasizes testing models for various psychiatric disorders for accuracy and evaluating treatment protocols for efficacy. Therapists' experiences in using the model have led to the refinement and expansion of the theoretical framework and to further protocols for the treatment of different disorders. Cognitive therapy continues to expand and evolve as a psychological treatment and in its conceptualization of psychopathology.

All cognitive therapies fundamentally assume that behavior is mediated by thoughts. Beck began to develop cognitive therapy because he observed that explanations for human behavior promulgated by psychoanalysts were less than satisfactory in accounting for what actually occurred in sessions with depressed patients. Conscious thoughts and the depressed patient's evaluation of his or her experience were observably negative and accessible for change. Similarly, behavior therapists (Mahoney, 1974) were noting that behavior therapy had limits in its capacity to explain and treat particular patients. At the same time that Beck was developing the cognitive therapy approach to depression, Seligman and Abramson (1979) were testing the theory that a negative explanatory style increased the risk for depression (see Chapter 9). In the form developed by Beck, cognitive therapy emphasizes current behavior and thoughts, and the therapist works to uncover the rules, values, and assumptions that a patient has developed over a lifetime and to evaluate and change any that would predispose the patient to an underlying disorder.

Each of the cognitively focused therapies has a particular theory that underscores psychopathology and a particular focus of change. They vary in the type of relationship the therapist has with the patient and the goals and structure of treatment. Several types are time-limited treatments with specific, goal-oriented outcomes—for example, stress inoculation training and problem-solving therapy. Those with more defined measurable outcomes are influenced more by earlier behavioral therapy treatments. All cognitive therapies emphasize educating the patient and share the central idea that the patient can minimize the impact of further episodes of dysfunction by employing the tools of therapy. All cognitive therapies share a philosophical position that emphasizes the capacity of human beings to control our beliefs and actions and that our emotions and actions are dependent on how we make meaning from our experience.

Mahoney and Ainkoff (1978) proposed a useful classification of the types of cognitive therapy, which organized it into three types. These included cognitive restructuring therapies, coping skills therapies, and problem-solving therapies. The main difference between the types is the degree to which the therapy works toward primarily cognitive or behavioral change.

Cognitive restructuring therapies have the basic philosophy that emotional pain and behavioral disturbance result from disturbances in thinking. They also help the patient learn to think more rationally and adaptively. Cognitive therapy, as defined by Beck, and Rational Emotive Behavior Therapy (REBT), developed by Albert Ellis, represent two paradigms with cognitive restructuring at the heart of therapy. REBT, another treatment assuming that human thinking, emotions, and behavior are interrelated, was developed at about the same time as cognitive therapy. It has not yet been as rigorously evaluated and thus has less support for its efficacy. Ellis developed a more general and philosophically based approach to psychotherapy. He proposed that all humans have common vulnerabilities to psychopathology—given their insufficient frustration tolerance and "shoulds," that is, irrational and illogical ideas that they have. The therapist in REBT works to directly influence the patient to change his belief system and behave more rationally (Dryden & Ellis, 2001).

Coping skills training therapies are treatments that involve training people to perform a set of skills that are designed to work better to help them cope with external situations that are stressful or that they find problematic. Thoughts are not specifically targeted unless they interfere with responding to the stressful event or exacerbate the person's negative response to the event. Examples of coping skills training include stress inoculation training (Meichenbaum, 1977) and systematic rational restructuring (Goldfried & Davison, 1976).

Problem-solving therapies have the goal of teaching the patient to employ a set of helpful strategies with a number of problematic situations. The strategies can be cognitive or behavioral. The therapist actively works with the patient to develop solutions to problems, with the assumption that this will lead to subsequent improvement in mood and behavior. D'Zurilla and Goldfried's (1976) problem-solving therapy and the subsequent applications by Nezu (2001) and others typify this approach.

REFERENCES

Butler, A. C., & Beck, J. S. (2000). Cognitive therapy outcomes: A review of meta-analyses. *Journal of the Norwegian Psychological Association, 37,* 1–9.

Dobson, K. S. (Ed.). (2001). *Handbook of cognitive-behavioral therapies* (2nd ed.). New York: The Guilford Press.

Dryden, W., & Ellis, A. (2001). Rational Emotive Behavior Therapy. In K. Dobson (Ed.), *Handbook of cognitive behavior therapies* (2nd ed., pp. 295–341). New York: The Guilford Press.

D'Zurilla, T. J., & Nezu, A. M. (2001). Problem-solving therapies. In K. Dobson (Ed.), *Handbook of cognitive behavior therapies* (2nd ed., pp 211–245). New York: The Guilford Press.

Goldfried, M. R., & Davison, G. C. (1976). *Clinical behavior therapy.* New York: Holt, Rinehart & Winston.

Mahoney. M. J. (1974). *Cognition and behavior modification.* Cambridge, MA: Ballinger.

Mahoney, M. J., & Ainkoff, D. B. (1978). Cognitive and self-control therapies. In S. L. Garfield & A. E. Bergin (Eds.), *Handbook of psychotherapy and behavioral change: An empirical analysis* (2nd ed., pp. 689–722). New York: Wiley.

Meichenbaum, D. H. (1977). *Cognitive–behavior modification.* New York: Plenum Press.

Seligman, M.E.P., Abramson, L.Y., Semmel, A., Vonbaeyer, C. (1979). Depressive attributional style. *Journal of Abnormal Psychology, 88,* 242–247.

Cognitive Model and Theory of Psychopathology

LEARNING OBJECTIVES

The reader will be able to:

1. Understand how cognitive therapy conceptualizes psychopathology.
2. Know the difference between automatic thoughts, intermediate beliefs, and core beliefs.
3. Understand the maintenance function of core beliefs.

Cognitive therapy conceptualizes psychopathology as derived from disturbances that occur in a patient's thinking. The cognitive model in its most basic form describes the connection between thoughts and emotion, behavior and physiology. Cognitive processes—that is, thoughts and the evaluation of perceptions—affect neural substrates and pathways in the central nervous system to produce emotional states and activate physiological reactions and behavior. Cognitive processes are affected by biology and, in turn, can alter neural pathways and neurotransmitter function. There are multiple recent studies that show the effects of cognitive therapy on the brain and biological systems; this is not surprising, since thoughts result from neurochemical interactions and the activation of neural pathways, and learning alters brain structure and function.

Consider the experience of being on a roller coaster—without the mediating thought that one was on a thrill ride—one's behavior, emotion, and physiology might be completely different when taking that 140-foot plunge. The initial global and biological response in such a situation—terror—is modified, reality tested, and corrected. So we think we are having fun and will pay extra for bigger scares. Social learning could influence our desire to take a ride as well ("everyone else is doing it"). Thus, individual perception, prior learning, development, and interpersonal influences color the meaning of an individual's experience. With time, selective attention to evidence can provide a strong basis for continual beliefs and patterns of interaction, whether or not they make logical sense or function effectively for us.

> **MR. WHITE** spends much of his time alone. When friends ask him to do things he thinks, "They just feel sorry for me." He feels irritated and sad and turns them down. Whenever Mr. White is in a social situation with a woman he is hypervigilant for signs of criticism. If she does not respond to something he says with an unequivocally positive remark he thinks, "I blew it." He feels sad and stops interacting with her.

As you can see, Mr. White's social interactions would be a source of anxiety and unhappiness rather than pleasure. While many of us would see an invitation to go out with friends as positive or as evidence of the pleasure our friends take in our company Mr. White's thought about this event is quite different. It is possible that neither our thought nor his is accurate. Mr. White thinks that the only reason that his friends want to spend time with him is because they pity him. The meaning of the irritation is more important to his subsequent reaction than the event itself. He has no evidence for his belief. His thought leads him to feel sad and angry and to behave in a way that will most probably ensure his getting fewer and fewer invitations. (People may respond to his repeatedly turning them down with the automatic thought "He's not interested in seeing us socially" and stop asking him.)

Additionally, were you to ask Mr. White how he felt after being in social situations with women, he would reply, "I feel like a failure," even though his feeling is sadness. It is common for patients and therapists to confuse thoughts and feelings with thoughts and facts. Patients will often say that the cause of unpleasant feelings is the situation and not the thoughts that they have about it. For example, if you ask Ms. Gray about why she cut herself, she will say "because I had a fight with my boyfriend."

The cognitive model of psychopathology asserts that psychopathological states share the idea that disturbances in thinking color perception in a particular way. For example, depressed patients generally think more negatively about themselves, others, and the future than the facts of their lives would indicate. These thoughts cause subsequent emotional, behavioral, and physiologic changes that produce symptoms and perpetuate psychopathology. Mr. White's reticence with women and constant scanning for criticism would make him a difficult person to get to know in a relationship and likely be frustrating to any potential partners. The result of his automatic thoughts and subsequent behavior would lead him to act in ways that produce the outcome that he believes—namely, that he does not measure up socially.

The disturbance in thinking underlying psychological disorders is organized by cognitive behavioral therapists into three categories. The first, automatic thoughts, can be about the self, the world, other people, and/or the future. These groups of thoughts, when negative in depressed patients, are known as the cognitive triad. Automatic thoughts arise spontaneously and are not consciously directed and when associated with psychological disturbance often produce dysphoric affect. Automatic thoughts are the easiest type of thoughts to change. In psychological disturbances automatic thoughts are frequently untrue or only partly true. Having the patient test automatic thoughts for accuracy frequently improves his or her symptoms.

Identifying automatic thoughts is a vital strategy used by cognitive therapists to help patients change. The technique used is to ask the patient what was going through his or her mind when he or she discusses a difficult situation or when the therapist notes a shift in affect during a session. After the patient becomes proficient in identifying thoughts the therapist teaches him or her methods to evaluate automatic thoughts associated with dysphoric affect for accuracy. This is done by evidence gathering, generating more plausible explanations, asking what the patient would tell a friend who had this thought, determining if the thought is really a problem to be solved, and so forth. Patients learn to generate plausible alternative explanations, rate how plausible they are, and rate the change in their emotional state that results from believing the alternative explanation. The aim is to help the patient reach more logical conclusions about evidence in the presence of strong negative affect and to demonstrate that reaching those conclusions has a helpful effect on the patient's mood and behavior.

MR. WHITE was instructed by his therapist to gather evidence that his friends had a genuine interest in him and did not "just feel sorry for him." Over time he was able to evaluate his relationships and use this information to see that although it was true that many of his friends were concerned about him since his breakup, they had also been interested in doing things with him socially before he broke up with his girlfriend. This realization allowed him to accept a few invitations, and when he went out he found that he felt much better.

Ultimately, the therapist works to determine what meanings a situation has for the patient, since understanding why events have certain meanings is what allows the patient and therapist to begin the process of understanding intermediate and core beliefs. This second group of thoughts is important to cognitive therapists as they organize their conceptualization of patients. These thoughts are best understood as the "rules" an individual has developed over time that lead both to expectations of himself or herself and others and guide behavior. Intermediate beliefs can also serve a second function—as protection from the core beliefs that a patient may have. For example, if a patient has a core belief, "I'm defective," he or she could develop an intermediate belief that "If I work to please everyone, I'll get by," in order to cope with this painful internal thought that he or she has about himself or herself.

MR. WHITE had the experience of being continually criticized by his mother. He also was ashamed of his birthmark and felt that people would criticize his physical appearance. He learned from a young age that "If people got close to me, they will be critical and know I'm defective." Because these thoughts were painful and developing relationships had the potential to reveal what he believed to be terrible weakness, he kept people at arm's length.

Finally, the groups of thoughts known as "core beliefs" or "schemas" are of significant importance to cognitive therapists. This is because, despite an emphasis on current thoughts and behavior in cognitive therapy, the modification of these beliefs is necessary to produce more enduring improvement. Understanding the development of these core beliefs is a fundamental feature in understanding a particular patient. Negative biases about oneself or other people make a person much more vulnerable to life stresses and events. In treating a patient with a personality disorder, core beliefs are frequently "activated," that is, close to the surface, and can present as the patient's automatic thoughts. When cognitive therapists talk about the activation of core beliefs, they are referring to a process where underlying basic and fundamental beliefs about the self, others, or the world are triggered by an internal or external event or mood state. These beliefs can be positive or negative, functional or dysfunctional. The beliefs worked on in cognitive therapy are generally negative and dysfunctional ones that have led to the development of behavioral strategies that are too costly or too painful for the patient to sustain.

Core beliefs generally remain unarticulated unless they are triggered or extremely negative or unless they are inquired about and explored in therapy. They are often learned early in life and are typically fairly rigid. Core beliefs are experienced as reality by a person, whether or not this is the case. They can often be the reason why neutral or somewhat aversive events can mean something devastating to the patient. For example, although divorce is stressful for everyone, for some patients the loss is devastating because of what it means about them as people—it activates core beliefs of being unlovable and worthless.

> **MR. WHITE** is having coffee with four friends from class. He makes a remark about a TV show that he saw. One of the women in the group looks away after he makes this remark and waves to another person across the room. He feels embarrassed and hurt, and his first thought is, "She must think I'm an idiot." Mr. White abruptly excuses himself and leaves the table.

The situation that activated this automatic thought is the woman waving to another friend following Mr. White's remark. His interpretation of this event is reflected in his automatic thought, "She must think I'm an idiot." This thought has no clear evidence for (or against) it, but Mr. White's subsequent affect and behavior are evidence of his strong and unquestioned belief that it is true. His behavior is likely to be noted by his friends as unusual (at the least). Mr. White, after further questioning in therapy, describes an underlying rule that if someone does not pay total attention to what he says, it is because they think he is stupid. A deeper rule he has is that if someone thinks he is stupid, it is intolerable; because it will mean that they have discovered the most fundamental negative belief that he holds about himself, that he is defective. Thus, his core belief, "I'm defective," is the most basic reason for the cascade of events.

Cognitive therapists believe that people develop an internal framework for structuring and making sense of their experience that is influenced by a number of different factors. These include genetics, temperament, early life experiences, relationships, trauma, culture, modeling, learning, and biology. No one factor is primary, all of them work together to affect how we make sense of the world.

MR. WHITE has developmental influences that have shaped much of his worldview. His mother criticized him, his father was absent, and he had no siblings that were models for alternative beliefs about his worth; he hardly knew his three oldest sisters. He saw the success of his younger sisters as meaning that they were capable and he was not; that he could never measure up. His stature and birthmark further added to his belief about himself as different and inferior, and culturally, this was reinforced, since small stature is often less preferred, particularly in boys. When his peers teased him, he felt completely defenseless and devastated. He withdrew from social interaction because he felt so anxious, leading to less attention from the adults in his life and fewer relationships with peers. His life experience gave him few models for other, more effective means of social interactions and more objective ways to evaluate himself in the world.

Core beliefs also play another important role in psychological development. These beliefs and the compensatory strategies a person develops can serve as a powerful maintenance and reinforcement function for distorted perceptions. This is one way that core beliefs are maintained over time, even when there is ample evidence that refutes them in a patient's history. For example, when one is a youngster and has a basic belief, "I'm incompetent," a person may develop a strategy of not trying any new behaviors or learning any new skills in order to avoid being exposed as being incompetent. The end result, however, is that one would miss the possibility of discovering that there were things that he or she could do effectively and one would develop skill deficits that would actually make him or her less effective.

Most people have a predominance of positive core beliefs and see themselves as basically effective and good. When individuals have selectively negative core beliefs that are painful (e.g., "I'm unlovable"), they develop a number of mitigating strategies and beliefs to lessen the possible effects of this belief (e.g., "If I take care of everyone and don't need much, I'll get by"), or not feel the resultant dysphoria. When these strategies fail or circumstances occur that cannot be mitigated by the strategy (e.g., breaking up with a significant other), the painful core belief can become predominant. The beliefs then function as a screen that filters and distorts information and events that the person encounters. A good example of a belief that functions like a core belief is prejudice. An individual who has a strong prejudice will discount or distort evidence that would, if noticed, serve to alter this belief. This individual's feelings and behavior toward a group of people are not determined by facts, but by how he or she structures these facts. An activated negative core belief can similarly influence an individual to process information so that he or she continues to strengthen negative perceptions and discounts alternative information.

When **MR. WHITE** broke up with his girlfriend, it served to activate his belief that he was socially inadequate and unlovable. Just as he did in childhood, he felt that it would be terrible if people knew this about him, and he began to compensate by withdrawing from social interactions. He began to do less and has had little contact with other people. When friends call him to go out, he thinks that they are "only doing it out of pity" and therefore turns them down. As they call him less and less frequently, given his constant refusal, he sees this as evidence of his not being capable of having social interactions or of making friends.

MS. GRAY consistently thinks of herself as worthless. When she spends time with friends and they talk about personal matters she will often "get crazy" and suggest that they "go out and party." These "parties" frequently result in her becoming intoxicated and then getting sexually involved with men she does not know. The next day, she feels more worthless and alienated from her friends. Because of her belief that if people really knew her they would not want to be her friend and her subsequent anxiety, she compensates by avoiding intimacy and suggesting they "party." Ms. Gray's drinking and sexual involvement with strangers perpetuate her feeling out of control and worthless.

Patients make efforts to avoid the activation of core beliefs by engaging in compensatory strategies or avoiding the situations that trigger these beliefs. Avoidance keeps problematic beliefs from being activated, but it also means that the beliefs cannot be refuted. Compensatory strategies are used by everyone, but overuse or exclusive use of less adaptive strategies like hypervigilance, worry, or self-destructive behavior, can cause self-fulfilling prophecies, as illustrated in the previous patient examples. In personality disorders, compensatory strategies are overused both because of how rigid and inflexible these strategies are in personality-disordered patients and because of the nearly constant activation of core beliefs. Patients with personality disorders also use less adaptive strategies because of skill deficits, like lack of assertiveness or emotion regulation skills. These deficits develop due to the early development of personality disorder and patients' inflexibility and overuse of compensatory strategies.

Learning points

- The fundamental premise of cognitive therapy is that thoughts directly affect emotion, behavior, and physiology.
- Automatic thoughts can be positive or negative, rational or irrational.
- Intermediate and core beliefs are how people derive the meaning of experiences and develop over time.
- Changing automatic thoughts to more accurate thoughts improves symptoms in psychological disturbances; changing intermediate and core beliefs produces more enduring improvement.

REFERENCES

Beck, J. S. (1995). *Cognitive therapy: Basics and beyond*. New York: The Guilford Press.

Goldapple, K. S., Segal, Z., Garson, C., et al. (2004). Modulation of cortical-limbic pathways in major depression: Treatment-specific effects of cognitive therapy. *Archives of General Psychiatry, 61,* 34–41.

Schwartz, J. M., & Begley, S. (2002). *The Mind and the brain: Neuroplasticity and the power of mental force*. New York: Harper Collins.

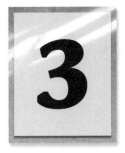

3

Case Formulation

LEARNING OBJECTIVES

The reader will be able to:

1. Understand case conceptualization according to a cognitive therapy framework.
2. Outline the particular features of a cognitive case conceptualization.
3. Recognize the features of the cognitive conceptualization that make the therapeutic approach unique to each patient.

In any system of psychotherapy a vital element is the conceptualization of the patient. This formulation seeks to account for four basic areas of information—predisposing factors for the disorder (Why me?), precipitating factors (Why now?), perpetuating factors (What keeps this problem going?), and protective factors (Why hasn't it gotten worse?). A particular theoretical framework also informs a formulation, that is, how the therapist thinks psychological disturbance happens and how he or she understands human development and interactions.

Cognitive therapists consider multiple determinants—biological, psychological, and social—as the factors that influence how a patient comes to structure his or her experience. Biological factors include genetics, temperament, internal and external biological influences (physical illness, medications, and substances), and innate biological predispositions (development of language and emotion). Psychological factors include modeling, conditioning, and trauma, as well as comparison and identification. Social influences include historical and cultural contexts, spiritual beliefs, and the effects of poverty and deprivation, which join with biological and psychological determinates to form the context for the development of an individual set of rules and beliefs that structures experience.

In cognitive therapy, the therapist considers the patient's personal and developmental history, the present problem and triggering events, and the automatic thoughts that the patient has in emotionally difficult situations and synthesizes these pieces of information in the context of the cognitive model for a particular disorder. A fundamental question to form a case conceptualization is to determine why a patient has been unable to implement his or her own solutions for a particular problem. The initial part of the formulation often involves a cross-section of the patient's thoughts, emotions, and behaviors in a particular situation and the resulting affects of these on the patient.

When **MS. GREEN** found out that her daughter was pregnant, she became excessively preoccupied with worries about her daughter's physical health and more worried about her own physical health and safety. One afternoon, while doing the laundry, she stood up rapidly and felt light-headed. Her first thought was that she might be having a stroke. She rapidly became anxious and began to scan herself for other physical symptoms. The initial thought that she could be having a stroke was quite believable to her and increased her anxiety. She started to breathe more rapidly as she felt more and more anxious. This overbreathing increased her light-headedness and the thought that something dreadful was happening. She began to experience chest pain and a sense that she could not get sufficient air. She felt more light-headed, had numbness and tingling in her fingers, and was even more convinced that she was experiencing a dreadful physical calamity. Eventually she had a full-blown anxiety attack; she phoned her sister, who came over, helped her to calm down, and gave her an alprazolam. Ms. Green thought, "That was close—I don't know what would have happened to me if my sister hadn't come to help." Ms. Green developed an enduring worry that if the panic attack happened again it might be even more dangerous.

Here, we begin to conceptualize this patient vignette by looking at two triggering events—the background of excessive worry and overconcern with physical health and the physical trigger provided by normal postural orthostatic blood pressure changes. This combination triggered the thought "I must be having a stroke" in Ms. Green, which a cognitive therapist would recognize as a catastrophic misinterpretation of body sensations, based on the knowledge he or she had about the cognitive model for panic disorder. This catastrophic misinterpretation, along with the probability distortions in Ms. Green's thinking (meaning her thoughts that bad things are more likely to happen to her than to other people), leads her to have an increase in the physiological symptoms of anxiety, to which she selectively attends. The physiological symptoms associated with anxiety augment with overbreathing and eventually she has a full-scale panic attack. Her subsequent behavior, calling her sister and getting medication, will be powerfully reinforced, as it will be associated with the cessation of such painful anxiety. In addition, her final thought, "that was close," would serve a powerful maintenance function; rather than learn that what happened to her was not dangerous, she interprets the situation as one where she was fortunate to escape further harm.

The conceptualization of Ms. Green's panic attack is an example of how a cognitive therapist conceptualizes a single instance of thoughts, emotions, behavior, and physiology triggered by a set of events and having a particular outcome. The interconnected nature of the cognitive model for panic disorder and how the model expresses itself in this particular patient is apparent, as is the crucial element of observing subsequent events and cognitions, and their maintenance and reinforcing function.

In terms of the cognitive model, cognitive therapists attempt to understand the patient, the behaviors that are currently a problem, and the problematic emotional and physiological states that are currently active. This usually involves identifying the automatic thoughts that are associated with and/or potentially maintaining problematic emotions or behaviors. The therapist also pinpoints the event(s) that triggers these thoughts. Frequently, the patient complains that this event is the cause of the problem. For example, Mr. White came to therapy because he had broken up with his girlfriend and he felt the breakup was the cause of his problem. Although most people would be sad at the ending of a relationship, only a small number of them would develop a major depression. The thoughts, emotions, and behaviors that follow the breakup, as well as the activation of his core belief and subsequent change in information processing, produce and maintain the psychological disturbance that follows. Once the patient learns to identify the automatic thoughts that relate to dysphoric states or dysfunctional behavior, those thoughts that are central to the problem are targeted for therapeutic intervention, and with the development and personal history of the patient, provide the foundation for the conceptualization.

In addition to understanding how the patient's automatic thoughts relate to the problem, the therapist also begins to evaluate and determine what processes perpetuate the particular disorder. Core beliefs and the strategies patients develop to deal with core beliefs (like avoidance, substance use, and worry) are often basic reasons for continuing problems. Skill deficits that remain uncorrected are often another perpetuating factor. If a patient believes the world is consistently depriving and has never learned to be assertive, this belief is likely to persist. Interpersonal and environmental conditions often perpetuate disorders—unrelenting stress can cause a person to consider things more absolutely and globally and decrease his or her capacity to logically solve problems and remember. Think about how inaccurately you appraise situations after several nights of poor or no sleep. Significant others can frequently punish a patient for effective and skillful behavior; as an example, a spouse may withdraw affection when a patient behaves in a more independent way.

The second level of the formulation involves identifying the patient's intermediate beliefs and beginning to develop hypotheses about his or her core beliefs. The therapist does this with a number of tools. First, he or she has learned about development, learning, biology, temperament, and culture and how these processes influence the attribution style of humans. Second, he or she has a particular developmental and interpersonal history of the patient and uses this to hypothesize about the origin and maintenance of the patient's core beliefs. Third, he or she has thought records that the patient brings to treatment that may have common themes. These themes often hold clues to the idiosyncratic vulnerability of the patient to psychological distress. The therapist can enlarge on these themes by asking the patient, "What does having the thought that you are _____ mean about you?" Another important technique is to pay attention to the patient's verbal and nonverbal behavior for affect shifts within a session that might signal the patient is relating thoughts that are closely linked to his or her intermediate and core beliefs. Finally, the therapist has reports of how the patient interacts with and has expectations of significant others in his or her life and has firsthand experience about how the patient behaves toward and thinks about the therapist.

 MS. GREEN brought in several thought records that described situations where she was called on to complete a task and became extremely anxious. In each situation she had the thought that she would fail to complete the task in an adequate way. The therapist asked her, "What would it mean about you if you didn't do (the task) exactly as you wanted?" She replied, "People will think I'm a failure." The therapist and Ms. Green agreed that a rule that governed her behavior was that if she were to do something that did not meet her standards it would mean to her that other people would see that she was a failure, and she would see herself as a failure as well. As therapy proceeded, the therapist and Ms. Green began to consider the question of what it would mean if people saw her as a failure at doing certain things, and she responded that it would mean that she had lost control. The therapist began to hypothesize that this thought, "I'm out of control," represented a core belief for Ms. Green.

MS. GRAY was able to complete thought records relatively easily. Nearly all of them had the automatic thought, "I'm bad," as the identified thought when she was dysphoric. Ms. Gray's therapist began to test the assumption that Ms. Gray had a core belief that she was bad, and that this belief was consistently activated by multiple events, and substantially strengthened by the strategies Ms. Gray had developed to deal with this belief, namely emotional avoidance and substance use. Her therapist carefully introduced the possibility that the idea that she was bad could seem real to her, given the early learning experiences she had. He explained that Ms. Gray's subsequent behavior and relationships would also strengthen the idea that she was bad, even though the idea might not be true. The therapist suggested that they might consider together a new belief that they could test that might describe Ms. Gray more accurately and be more functional even if it didn't "feel" true just now. Ms. Gray said that she could not imagine another idea about herself.

Patients with personality disorders often have constant activation of their core beliefs by external events. The therapist working with a patient who has a personality disorder often needs to provide a more functional belief to the patient, and collaboratively design ways for the patient to gather evidence both for and against a more functional and accurate view of himself or herself. The therapist also tries to understand and mitigate the maintenance of the old core belief by compensatory strategies. The therapist helps the patient to correct skill deficits and to develop more flexible responses to negative perceptions and emotional states.

Conceptualization is collaborative in cognitive therapy. This means that after the therapist forms an initial hypothesis he or she shares it with the patient and they work together to refine and expand an understanding of how the problem came to be. This experience can be powerful because patients see that there is a different way to understand the nature and development of their problems, and therefore have the capacity to generate solutions. Collaboratively conceptualizing the patient's problems implies an understanding that the problems are manageable and make sense in the context of the patient's life experience. The therapist teaches the patient how developmental events influenced how the patient learned about the world and himself or herself, and importantly, how the strategies that the patient used to cope perpetuated and strengthened his or her beliefs. The therapist notes the assets and positive coping mechanisms of the patient and helps him or her to strengthen and use these attributes to tackle problems and cope with adversity. A profound strengthening of the therapeutic alliance is often the result of collaborating with the patient to understand a different framework for how his or her problems came to be. Often what has seemed inexplicable and shameful takes on a new and more hopeful meaning as the patient looks with an alternative perspective at why and how he or she has reached this point in life.

As **MS. GREEN** worked in therapy, she and her therapist considered several factors that contributed to her terror about losing control. First, she described being a child who was always anxious about pleasing other people; her father was prone to angry outbursts and Ms. Green was terrified of him. She was always the child who was able to calm him down and was often sent by her mother to talk with him after he got home from work, when no one in the family knew what to expect him to do. Ms. Green had a great deal of apprehensiveness about new situations throughout her childhood. She remembers her family saying that she was "always like that." Ms. Green was responsible for the care of her siblings at a young age and was extremely anxious about failing in her duties and the children coming to harm. She developed the strategy of working and reworking tasks to avoid any scrutiny and to make certain that she would not make any mistakes. She rarely had experiences that would allow her to find out that mistakes were not dangerous, because she always turned in "perfect" homework and school projects. The therapist also hypothesized that her chronic overconcern for her family and worry stemmed from her belief that she was somehow protecting herself and others by worrying, and the patient confirmed that she had learned this way of dealing with problems by watching her mother's behavior. Finally, Ms. Green had been molested by a neighbor. This experience terrified her and left her with the lifelong idea that she had been responsible. She believed that only by being constantly vigilant could she ever avoid an event that was this overwhelming.

Data that the therapist gathers from therapeutic impasses can be an important part of the conceptualization. Disruptions of the therapeutic alliance, failure of the patient to do homework, and problems that resist reasonable solutions can furnish the therapist and patient with the opportunity to explore the underlying beliefs and rules that interfere with the patient's life and add to the conceptual framework.

MS. GREEN refused to do thought records as her therapist requested. She initially told him she "didn't have time" because of her household responsibilities. After a thorough explanation of the importance of homework and problem solving to help her to find time, Ms. Green still did not complete the thought records. Finally, the therapist asked her "what went through her mind" as she thought about doing the homework. She said, "I'll screw it up, and you'll think I'm a complete idiot." Further exploration of this allowed the therapist to understand the role perfectionism played in Ms. Green's life.

By developing an individual case conceptualization, cognitive therapists can plan treatment that is specifically focused on the needs of a particular patient. Ms. Green not only requires exposure and cognitive restructuring as regards her physical symptoms of panic, but she also needs to correct her misconception about worry and to become more comfortable with making mistakes and with feeling uncertainty. Her treatment must help her to understand the affects of being molested, to allow her to appropriately grieve and be angry about that experience, and to develop a more realistic appraisal of her neighbor being responsible for this unfortunate event. Ms. Green must learn to monitor herself for fears of loss of control and to evaluate how logical those fears are.

A number of excellent tools exist for therapists to use to help guide their thinking as they begin the process of conceptualization. Judith Beck's book, *Cognitive Therapy: Basics and Beyond,* includes both a written case format and a conceptualization diagram that can help to organize the therapist's data. The Academy of Cognitive Therapy provides a format for case conceptualization and an example of a written case conceptualization, which are included in the appendix.

Learning points

- Individual case conceptualization is a critical component of cognitive therapy.
- The therapist conceptualizes patients by looking at particular instances of thoughts, emotions, and behavior and then identifying patterns that synthesize these with the patient's developmental history, the patient's current circumstance, and the cognitive model for the disorder.
- Patients with personality disorders have more complex conceptualizations that often require discussion of developmental issues and core beliefs early in therapy.

REFERENCES

Beck, J. S. (1995). *Cognitive therapy: Basics and beyond.* New York: The Guilford Press.

Needleman, L. D. (1999). *Cognitive case conceptualization: A guidebook for practitioners.* Mashwah, NJ: Lawrence Erlbaum Associates.

Persons, J. B. (1989). *Cognitive therapy in practice: A case formulation approach.* New York: Norton.

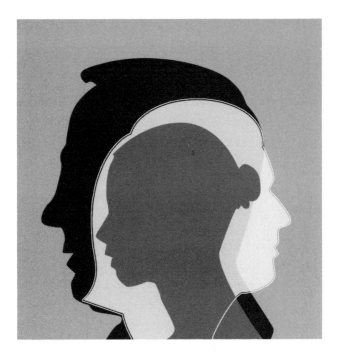

The Therapeutic Process and the Therapeutic Relationship in Cognitive Therapy

The Patient–Therapist Relationship

LEARNING OBJECTIVES

The reader will be able to:

1. Define collaborative empiricism.
2. Understand the stance of the therapist in cognitive behavioral therapy.
3. Learn how transference and countertransference are defined and used in cognitive behavioral therapy.

The cornerstone of the relationship between the therapist and patient in cognitive therapy is collaborative empiricism—a term coined by Beck, Rush, Shaw, and Emery in 1979. The relationship is characterized as one where two investigators work together to evaluate data for accuracy. Both the therapist and patient assume an equally active stance in helping the patient to solve his or her problems. The aim is for the patient to consider himself or herself a scientist and to objectively and rationally consider his or her thoughts, emotions, and behavior. This requires the patient to think in a logical way, to view his or her own thinking as not necessarily accurate, and to accept the premise that his or her thoughts are associated with his or her symptoms. Helping the patient to become a coinvestigator is not always easy. Many patients do not come to treatment thinking that their thoughts, rules, and beliefs are hypotheses to be tested and that the therapist's role is to be inquisitive, active, and directive. Cognitive therapists recognize that developing a strong therapeutic alliance with collaborative empiricism as a central focus is essential for a good therapeutic outcome.

 MS. GRAY was upset when she first started therapy. She came to her first session after intake and immediately began to talk about the fight she had had with a friend, her irresponsible boyfriend, the problem she had with a teacher at school, and her feeling that she "just couldn't take it anymore." She became angry with the therapist when he tried to stop her for a moment to explain how they were going to work together. She said, "Your job is to let me vent; that's what therapists do." Gently, and deliberately, the therapist explained that although he wanted to hear about and acknowledge her distress and understand her problems, it was important that Ms. Gray understand that therapy would involve not just his listening, but the two of them working together to understand, evaluate, and change the thoughts, emotions, and behaviors she had.

Several features of the structure of cognitive therapy treatment facilitate the development of an active and collaborative relationship. These include the empathic stance of the therapist, the structuring of sessions, and the mandate to provide as much information as possible to the patient—about his or her illness, the conceptualization of his or her current problems, and the treatment itself. The therapist can educate the patient directly, and print material and Web sites can augment this education. Therapists can increase collaboration with the patient by explaining the rationale for interventions in a detailed way. A common misconception is that cognitive therapy is one size fits all; that is, that treatment proceeds by a formula without considering the individual needs of the patient. Treatment, and the therapist's approach to the patient, is tailored specifically to provide efficient and effective symptom relief and problem solving.

An open, warm, and active stance is optimal for the cognitive behavioral therapist. The beginning therapist should be well grounded in basic relationship skills common to all good psychotherapy—warmth, genuineness, empathy, professionalism, and active listening. He or she must be skilled at setting limits and maintaining boundaries in treatment. The therapist must make certain that rapport with the patient is strong and he or she must consistently attend to the therapeutic alliance. He or she must be particularly flexible when working with personality-disordered patients. An important fact for the therapist to remember when working with patients who have personality disorders and assessing the strength of the alliance is that the patient may be missing fundamental adaptive relationship skills that need to be identified by the therapist as an important goal to learn in treatment.

MS. GRAY came to session complaining about a teacher at school who was "unfair and hateful." The therapist determined that the problem Ms. Gray had in class was that she often did not understand what the teacher meant when she assigned homework. For example, when the teacher asked the class to bring in a summary of the text, Ms. Gray would bring in a one- or two-line paper and be graded poorly. Ms. Gray had never asked the teacher for extra time or to explain what she meant by the assignment. She would be furious about the grades she received and would see the teacher as "bad and unfair." When the therapist asked Ms. Gray if she had ever considered asking the teacher to explain assignments further, she said, "No." Furthermore, when the therapist had Ms. Gray engage in a role-play where he was the teacher, Ms. Gray had no capacity to ask in a direct, clear, and assertive way for what her responsibility was for homework. The therapist switched roles, modeled being more assertive for Ms. Gray, and then asked her to practice this type of communication. Furthermore, the therapist asked Ms. Gray to specifically inform him if she didn't understand something in therapy and asked her at each session for feedback or questions about her understanding of the session. In this way, Ms. Gray got to practice being more assertive in a less threatening situation.

Cognitive therapists must be flexible and goal oriented. Striking the right balance of activity and listening is often difficult for novice therapists—particularly when they believe that what therapists do that is helpful is to listen and to allow patients to vent. The right balance of questions and therapist feedback reinforces an increase in the patient's activity and furthers participation in a collaborative relationship. Support in cognitive therapy comes from the fact that the therapist and patient work together to help solve the patient's problems, not just talk about them. Good therapists validate the patient's difficulties and help to make sense of them. Throughout, the therapist must be aware of the reactions that the patient is having to therapy. The therapist obtains direct verbal feedback about the session and is sensitive to patients' verbal and nonverbal responses within the session. This feedback informs the therapist about modifications and interventions necessary to ensure that the patient remains an engaged and active participant.

After the first several sessions, **MR. WHITE** came to therapy and said little. The therapist noted that he had been more depressed that week and that his Beck Depression Inventory (BDI) scores had increased. She became much more active in helping him to problem solve about a difficult work situation, as well as reassuring him that mood fluctuations were common during the first part of treatment for depression. Mr. White then told his therapist that his most significant fear was that "therapy wouldn't work." The therapist calmly asked him if he had any evidence that that would be the case, and he said, "It just seemed hopeless." The therapist explained to him that hopelessness was a common feeling in depression, and that there was good evidence that depressions like his responded well to cognitive therapy. She also told him that other options existed (like medication) to treat his depression if therapy did not work, and that together they would monitor his symptoms and decide what was needed. She asked Mr. White if he was willing to do an activity schedule as an experiment and increase his pleasurable activities in the next week to see if he would feel better. He agreed to try this. His mood improved, and therapy continued.

Treatment begins with establishing the relationship and educating the patient. In the first several sessions after assessment, the therapist presents a conceptual model to the patient about how he or she understands the patient's problems. This serves several purposes: it begins to educate the patient about the cognitive model; it starts the process of translating practical problems into psychological ones; and it strengthens the therapeutic alliance by helping the patient feel less alone and more understood by a genuinely concerned person who has a new view of how these problems came to be. The therapist explains the nature of cognitive therapy itself during many of the early sessions. An open discussion about what the patient expected treatment to be like and how he or she expected his or her problems to be solved can facilitate this process. A discussion about the nature of therapy is important because it allows the therapist to set the stage for the type of relationship that is optimal and for the active approach that the patient must take to observe his or her thoughts and behavior and solve problems. The patient's expectations also teach the therapist about what the patient knows about cognitive therapy and can provide information about how demoralized he or she is from contending with his or her difficulties.

The therapist consistently works in therapy to elicit and provide feedback to the patient. The therapist and patient monitor progress toward reaching attainable goals. Feedback and assessing the progress of therapy is a critical part of the therapist's role. It is especially important for the therapist to actively elicit negative feedback about the therapist or his or her interventions, and to make certain the patient has a clear understanding about the treatment. Patients do not readily engage in activities they do not see as helpful, so obtaining feedback may increase homework compliance and deepen the alliance.

MS. GRAY had not completed an activity schedule assigned by the therapist. On three occasions, she told the therapist that the assignment "was too hard." The therapist asked Ms. Gray to complete it with him in the session. When they began this process, Ms. Gray became furious, saying that the therapist "just wanted to make her look stupid." She also accused the therapist of being incompetent, since no other therapist had ever required her to do homework, and she believed that the therapist should "cure" her by having her "vent" in the session. The therapist patiently explained the rationale for homework and asked Ms. Gray if her other therapy sessions had helped her. When she said, "not much," he asked if she would consider doing homework as an experiment and she grudgingly agreed.

Cognitive therapists understand that most humans want to appear compliant. People commonly wish to appear as though they comprehend something that is being said, even when they don't. This process occurs even more often in situations where the role expectations are unequal—as in the relationship between therapist and patient. The stance of the therapist, therefore, is one that includes asking about problems with adherence (rather than about whether the patient has been adherent to a treatment regimen) and asking the patient to explain his or her understanding of a concept in his or her own words. Furthermore, the therapist can accept some responsibility for therapeutic tasks that do not go well; for example, if a patient does not complete a homework assignment, the therapist might evaluate with the patient whether his or her explanation of the assignment was appropriate. Since anxiety and depression frequently interfere with learning the therapist cannot be certain if his or her instructions and explanations have been understood without getting feedback from the patient. Summarizing, or having the patient summarize, the main points discovered or taught within a session is a routine part of the session. Summaries and feedback increase the level of trust and understanding in the relationship. Finally, feedback that the patient gives to the therapist provides information about the patient's rules and beliefs about other people (the therapist) and further helps the therapist conceptualize the patient.

After **MS. GREEN'S** second therapy session, the therapist asked her how she felt about the session and what she had learned. Ms. Green said that she felt terrible, but that it "wasn't the therapist's fault." He asked her what thoughts she had when she felt terrible. Ms. Green said, "I'm sure you know how stupid I am." The therapist explained that it was common for people to feel vulnerable and exposed when they first began to talk about themselves in therapy. He noted in his own mind that Ms. Green might be prone to feeling "stupid" when she talked about herself.

Despite the open and collaborative stance of the therapist, there may be instances when the patient misperceives the therapist consistent with his or her misperceptions of other people. Cognitive therapists call this transference. It is addressed directly by the therapist when the patient's view of the therapist interferes with treatment. Generally, transference is not addressed when the therapeutic alliance is strong and the patient's thoughts about the therapist are not interfering with the progress of treatment. If the patient has the expectation that the therapist is a professional who is interested in and capable of being helpful, the relationship will usually unfold with ease. Unfortunately, many people come to therapy with different beliefs and expectations about care providers. These beliefs can originate in beliefs about psychiatry and psychotherapy (sometimes stemming from prior treatment failures), from ideas about the meaning of mental illness, or from early experiences and subsequent expectations about care-taking figures. Some patients may experience the structure of the cognitive therapy treatment session as too rigid and depriving.

When a negative transference exists the therapist can directly discuss with the patient how overgeneralization of the patient's past experience may have led to the development of an inaccurate view of the therapist and treatment. Socratic questioning and examining evidence about the therapist and his or her behavior can be used to help the patient to recognize distortions in his or her thinking. Negative transference is extremely valuable information to the therapist. It provides direct access to patients' beliefs about other people and can be a source of direct and significant learning.

MR. WHITE came to his therapy session 20 minutes late. He was visibly irritated and not forthcoming about what he wanted to discuss on the agenda. The therapist asked about his homework assignment and Mr. White snapped that he found it "impossible." Further inquiry into his automatic thoughts about not completing his homework revealed that he was unable to understand the assignment and was convinced that the therapist would criticize him for this. Mr. White said he felt extremely angry because he was paying for therapy and did not want to pay someone to criticize him. The therapist tabled other agenda items in order to repair this breech of the therapeutic relationship. Together, she and Mr. White looked at the evidence he had to believe that the therapist would criticize him. They conceptualized this belief as typical of his expectations of other people, and understood it in view of what he learned from his mother's behavior. The therapist would, in later sessions, look at the consequences of Mr. White's overgeneralization about other people being critical of him, and the behavior and affects that followed this belief. She also kept in mind the possibility that Mr. White could overuse irritability as a defensive strategy to compensate when he felt that someone was being critical of him and made note of this in her conceptualization.

Emotions that are generated in therapy and the nature of the therapeutic relationship in itself can activate maladaptive beliefs in patients. This can be positive for patient change; Beck, et al. (1979) recognized that the therapist would have maximal impact when he or she works with a cognition associated with a substantial amount of emotion (so-named "hot cognitions"). When these highly charged cognitions occur about the therapist, it is a tremendous opportunity to affect change. Therapists must take advantage of these opportunities to step back with the patient and understand the situation in a wider context—considering the facts about the situation and the origins of these distorted ideas. Clues that maladaptive beliefs may have been generated in session include strong emotion, anxiety, nonverbal communication, not staying on a topic, not working with the therapist to problem solve, and procedural resistance (see Chapter 7).

MS. GREEN was prone to lengthy silences during the first weeks of therapy. She was visibly uncomfortable during these silent periods. The therapist made many empathic and validating statements, instructed her about the tasks of therapy, and asked for feedback about the sessions. This was not helpful. Finally the therapist asked directly what was going on in her mind during the silences in therapy. Ms. Green said she was worrying, and specifically that she would say the "wrong thing" to the therapist. The therapist used Socratic questioning and determined that Ms. Green used worry to avoid the feeling of anxiety that she experienced when she talked about herself with another person. The therapist asked her what danger there would be in talking about herself, and she said, "If I let someone get close to me they'll hurt me." The therapist began to develop the hypothesis that Ms. Green had core beliefs that included helplessness and vulnerability. Ms. Green and the therapist agreed that the pattern that she had of not letting people get close to her was one that would be useful to change. Ms. Green was assigned the task of gradually increasing self-revealing statements in therapy and examining her automatic thoughts and the therapist's behavior in response to these revelations. She was instructed to identify increases in worry about saying the wrong thing as a signal that she was anxious about the therapist getting too close. Eventually, she and the therapist were able to understand this reaction as being linked to her prior history of sexual abuse.

MS. GRAY and her therapist discussed the problems that she was having getting along with her roommates. Specifically, she would become enraged whenever they did not do things that she thought they should do—like include her in their social plans or check in with her when they were going to the store to ask if she needed anything. Ms. Gray shut herself in her bedroom with the music turned up and the lights off when she was enraged. She felt worthless and unloved. On occasion, she would cut herself, particularly if no one came to check on her. Ms. Gray's therapist role-played the situation with Ms. Gray to help her understand the point of view of her roommates; they certainly couldn't read her mind, and they needed more direct communication from her to interact in a more functional way. Ms. Gray flew into a rage, yelling at the therapist, "Now you are accusing me of being manipulative just like everyone else does!" She stood up and made for the door. At this point the therapist stopped her and asked her to sit down so that they could talk about what happened. The therapist worked to repair the alliance by calmly and curiously commenting on the sudden change in Ms. Gray's mood. The therapist said he was not aware how difficult and painful it was for Ms. Gray to look at this situation without becoming angry and upset and explained that he thought it would be helpful to investigate the thoughts she had about him in talking about the situation.

Countertransference in cognitive therapy is conceptualized as automatic thoughts and subsequent emotions that the therapist has about the patient. These automatic thoughts commonly have two sources: those that do not have a logical basis and stem from the therapist's own core beliefs, or those thoughts that stem from actual problems the therapist is having with the patient that he or she has failed to solve. The therapist can use his or her own automatic thought records to help to understand the nature of these thoughts and to find more rational ways of dealing with the problem. The therapist can identify what the patient is doing that poses a problem for the therapist, understand the origin and functional value of this behavior for the patient, and determine if it is a problem for the patient in his or her relationship with other people. It may be then possible to point out to the patient that there is an advantage to changing this behavior. Alternatively, the therapist may discover that working with a particular patient has activated a maladaptive core belief of his or her own and resolve this appropriately.

MR. WHITE'S therapist, a resident in psychiatry, found that she was extremely reluctant to confront his not completing homework. She knew that he avoided assignments in school because he had a fear of criticism. Despite this, she had the persistent thought, "I must be doing this incorrectly; if I gave him the right assignment, he'd do the homework." Using a thought record helped her to understand how her unrealistic expectations were keeping her from identifying a significant pattern in the patient, and she became more direct with Mr. White.

MS. GRAY was calling her therapist two or three times daily at the start of treatment. The precipitant for each of these calls was that she had become angry or anxious and wanted to cut or hurt herself. These calls could occur at any time of the day or night. The therapist told Ms. Gray in the first session that it was unacceptable to him that she hurt herself in any way and that if she felt the need to do so she should call. After 2 weeks of telephone calls, the therapist hung the telephone up at 3 A.M. and thought, "I need to transfer this patient; I can't be helpful to her; she's a borderline." In the clearer light of morning, the therapist realized that what he needed to do was praise Ms. Gray for not hurting herself and for using him as a resource. He needed to discuss with Ms. Gray that the frequency of her telephone calls was not allowing him to do his best work with her. Together, they would need to find a way for her to use other resources and to solve the problem of her need to speak to someone urgently in a way that would allow him to work with other patients, get adequate rest, and allow her to get the support she needed.

Evaluating the accuracy of case conceptualization for what is missing or what has been incompletely understood is also a helpful way to work to understand the patient and one's own response. Therapists can often gain further insight by obtaining supervision or consultation with a skilled colleague. If the therapist has dysfunctional thoughts about patients because of limited experience with a particular disorder or a failure to adequately set limits consultation can be particularly helpful.

Learning points

- The relationship between the patient and therapist in cognitive therapy is one that encourages the collaboration of two investigators working together to evaluate data. Trust and empathy are essential.
- The therapist must attend to educating the patient, providing feedback and summaries, and seeking feedback from the patient—both obvious and subtle.
- Transference and countertransference in cognitive therapy are considered the automatic thoughts that the patient has about the therapist, or the therapist about the patient, that need to be examined and corrected if they are not consistent with the goals of treatment.

REFERENCES

Beck, A. T., Rush, A. J., Shaw, B. F. et al. (1979). *Cognitive therapy of depression.* New York: The Guilford Press.

Beck, J. S. (1995). *Cognitive therapy: Basics and beyond.* New York: The Guilford Press.

Leahy, R. (1996). *Cognitive therapy: Basic principles and applications.* Northvale, NJ: Jason Aronson.

Tools of Treatment

LEARNING OBJECTIVES

The reader will be able to:

1. Learn the therapeutic approaches to evaluating automatic thoughts and problem solving.
2. Define guided discovery.
3. Employ behavioral methods to help patients.

Cognitive therapy is fundamentally problem-solving therapy. The therapist helps the patient to specify problems that are interfering with his or her life and forms hypotheses as to why the patient is not solving these problems on his or her own. The deficits patients have are generally a combination of skill deficits and motivational deficits. When problems are complex, the therapist must work to determine what the patient needs to change first to effectively move forward. Patients with personality disorders may appear to have far more skills than they actually do; when, in fact, they are looking to the interpersonal environment to provide them with cues as to how to behave. Relationships can also interfere with patients using skills that they have by punishing or not reinforcing effective and adaptive behavior.

MS. GREEN comes to her therapy session and is visibly upset. Her homework assignment had been to spend an hour each day practicing controlled breathing and relaxation. Each time she started a practice session,

> her husband would knock at the bedroom door to tell her that one of her daughters was calling or to ask her to help him to find something in the house. Ms. Green was at a loss as to how to handle this problem. The therapist had her role-play the situation with her husband. She was unable to assertively ask him to stop interrupting her in the role play. She told the therapist that she never asked for any privacy at home.

Here we have an example of a skill deficit—namely, a lack of knowledge as to how to behave in an assertive way—that would contribute to Ms. Green's problems. Her family has a long history of interacting with her in a way that makes her the caretaker in every interaction and reinforces her pattern of being nonassertive. Her husband is accustomed to her availability at any given moment, and his response to her need for privacy and time for herself may be to sabotage her efforts, whether he is aware of this or not.

> **MS. GRAY'S** mother called her to "check in" nearly every day. Ms. Gray liked talking to her mother—she felt "connected" and enjoyed the contact. Whenever Ms. Gray was feeling better and not having difficulty with getting along with other people or with feeling suicidal, her mother stopped calling. Ms. Gray would often be anxious that her mother was mad at her and begin to feel worse.

This example shows how interpersonal behavior can reinforce less skillful and maladaptive behavior in the patient and result in motivational deficits toward implementing more skilled and functional behaviors. Ms. Gray's mother inadvertently selectively attends to Ms. Gray feeling suicidal or having interpersonal difficulty, and withdraws reinforcement when Ms. Gray is behaving in a more skillful way. This pattern often happens with patients who have chronic interpersonal disturbances. Patients with borderline personality, for example, are often only attended to by the mental health system after extreme behavior (suicide attempts) and not when they are attempting to call or get help at other times. Motivational deficits can also occur because of the specific effects of psychopathology; if you are depressed, and the depression has made you think that things are hopeless, you will not try as hard to alter your situation. Beliefs about change can also alter the potential to be motivated to try new things; if you have a basic belief that "people never change," or "change is dangerous," your capacity to try things differently will be limited.

The therapist, in collaboration with the patient, defines what existing problems require solutions. This process begins by setting goals with the patient at the start of treatment. These goals should be as specific and measurable as possible and put in behavioral terms. When a patient is particularly hopeless, the therapist may need to work at generating a partial list of goals by using Socratic questioning (e.g., asking the patient how he or she spent time before having the problems that he or she is having now; asking what the patient would be accomplishing if he or she was feeling like himself or herself). The therapist must carefully evaluate the goals that the patient defines, often by breaking them into manageable parts, to make certain that they are reasonably attainable. The therapist needs to acquire the skill to determine the difference between practical problems that the patient has and psychological problems that interfere with the patient's ability to solve practical matters. This distinction is a vital part of the case conceptualization and often evolves over several sessions as the therapist gathers data about the patient. After the list is generated, the therapist prioritizes the problems and together with the patient starts the process of problem solving. The patient and therapist should use the goals defined to guide treatment and evaluate progress.

When **MS. GREEN** came to treatment and her therapist asked her what she would like to change in therapy, she said that her goal was to "feel better." The therapist did not stop there; he asked specific questions about what feeling better would mean and what Ms. Green would be doing differently were she to be recovered. Together they generated a list of goals including having fewer panic attacks, being able to leave the house alone and to take public transportation, worrying for a shorter time period during the day, and developing a more assertive and direct method of communicating with other people. She and her therapist will add to the goal list as therapy proceeds.

Patients are often unaware of the steps involved in solving a problem, and even therapists, who may be innately skilled at this process, sometimes do not think about the mechanisms involved. First, the therapist works with the patient to generate solutions. Brainstorming, that is, rapidly generating a series of possible solutions without evaluation or judgment, is a great tool to use. Brainstorming often empowers patients to be far more creative and access abilities and solutions they ignore because of automatic thoughts about performance. The next step is to assess which solution is most desirable to try first by evaluating the advantages/disadvantages of each. The therapist helps the patient to choose the most workable solution, obtains a commitment, and makes a plan for him or her to implement that solution. The therapist and patient evaluate the results. Frequently, living with psychiatric disturbances produces tangible, resolvable problems that require attention (e.g., at work, in relationships). The patient's thoughts about these types of problems can reflect an accurate need for alternative behaviors and solutions. Cognitive therapy does not seek to put a positive spin on negative events—realistic thinking is what is sought. Accurate empathy about the real problems that confront many patients is a critical element of nurturing the therapeutic alliance and helping the patient to be motivated to try new behaviors.

As **MS. GREEN** became less anxious and more assertive, her conflicts with her husband became more frequent. He began drinking, a problem which he had had in the past, but which had been less of an issue recently. He accused Ms. Green of not taking care of the household properly and demanded that she pay better attention to him or he would leave her. Ms. Green's therapist spent time in session empathically discussing how difficult it must be for Ms. Green to face what she saw as the choice of contending with this significant rift in her marriage or returning to her previous style of relating to her husband. Instead of taking an either/or approach to the problem, the therapist helped her to generate options for contending with the conflict and to empathize with her husband's point of view. The therapist helped her to recognize how difficult it is to make a change of this magnitude, that some of the obstacles she faced were real, and that she could work to generate solutions.

The most fundamental therapeutic tool employed by cognitive therapists is the automatic thought record. This basic and valuable resource helps patients to notice and record the thoughts they have in the presence of strong, unpleasant affect and guides them to respond to their thinking in more rational and functional ways. Thought records can make the patient's emotions understandable because they occur in the context of his or her thinking—feelings no longer seem to come out of the blue. The patient recognizes that he or she is not at the mercy of external events or his or her emotions. The thought record also can point out the antecedents and consequences of behavior and can be useful to help the patient control triggers for more dysfunctional behavior. An example of a dysfunctional thought record can be found in Figure 5-1.

Directions: When you notice your mood getting worse, ask yourself, "What's going through my mind right now?" and as soon as possible jot down the thought or mental image in the Automatic Thought column.

Date/time	Situation	Automatic thought(s)	Emotions(s)	Adaptive response	Outcome
	1. What actual event or stream of thoughts, or daydreams or recollection led to the unpleasant emotion? 2. What (if any) distressing physical sensations did you have?	1. What thought(s) and/or image(s) went through your mind? 2. How much did you believe each one at the time?	1. What emotion(s) (sad/anxious/angry/ etc.) did you feel at the time? 2. How intense (0–100%) was the emotion?	1. (optional) What cognitive distortion did you make? 2. Use questions at bottom to compose a response to the automatic thought(s). 3. How much do you believe each response?	1. How much do you now believe each automatic thought? 2. What emotion(s) do you feel now? How intense (0–100%) is the emotion? 3. What will you do (or did you do)?
Friday 3/8 3 P.M.	Thinking about asking Bob if he wants to have coffee.	He won't want to go with me. 90%	Sad. 75%	(Fortune—telling error) I don't really know if he wants to or not. (90%) He is friendly to me in class. (90%) The worst that'll happen is he'll say no and I'll feel bad for a while. (90%) The best is he'll say yes. (100%) The most realistic is he may say yes but still act friendly. (80%) If I keep on assuming he doesn't want to go out with me, I'll have no chance with him. (100%) I should just go up and ask him. (50%) What's the big deal anyway? (75%)	1. A.T—50% 2. Sad—50% Anxious—50%

Questions to help compose an alternative response: (1) What is the evidence that the automatic thought is true? Not true? (2) Is there an alternative explanation? (3) What's the worst that could happen? Could I live through it? What's the best that could happen? What's the most realistic outcome? (4) What's the effect of my believing the automatic thought? What could be the effect of my changing my thinking? (5) What should I do about it? (6) If _____ (friend's name) were in the situation and had this thought, what would I tell him/her?

FIGURE 5-1 ■ Dysfunctional Thought Record. Copyright 1995 by Judith S. Beck, Ph. D. Reprinted with permission from *Cognitive Therapy: Basics and Beyond.* New York: The Guilford Press. 1995.

The therapist teaches the patient to fill out the dysfunctional thought record, generally during at least two sessions. The skill required to identify and change automatic thoughts is difficult for many patients, and therapists must be patient and deliberate in teaching each part of the process. The first task involves teaching the patient the cognitive model, generally by using an example from the patient's life in the last week. The therapist and patient complete the first part of a thought record together in the session so that the therapist is certain that the patient has the skill. The therapist teaches the patient to identify automatic thoughts by asking, "What just went through your mind?" when the patient is describing an emotionally upsetting situation or when the therapist notes a negative affect in the session.

MS. GREEN and her therapist began the work of understanding how her thoughts related to her problems. He explained what an automatic thought is—an image or thought that occurs just outside of awareness unless one focuses attention on the thought. He explained that these appraisals of events go on all the time, and that on occasion, they can be associated with strong emotions and can engender behavioral and physiological responses. He illustrated this by helping Ms. Green recount a time when she had a bout of indigestion after a Mexican dinner and thought, "I ate too much spicy food." She had a completely different reaction than when she had indigestion for which she had no explanation. Her automatic thought when she had indigestion without having had Mexican food was, "This could be a sign of something serious—I could be having a heart attack." This catastrophic thought produced different emotional and physiological reactions. The therapist explained the usefulness of evaluating automatic thoughts for accuracy to Ms. Green. He said that the first step was to collect her thoughts. He taught Ms. Green to ask herself the question, "What just went through my mind?" whenever she had a strong emotion, and to note the situation, her automatic thought, and her emotional response at that time.

Therapists can use imagery and role-play, as well as to ask the patient directly, to help the patient to identify automatic thoughts. The patient who is having trouble identifying automatic thoughts can also become more proficient if the therapist asks him or her if he or she is thinking something opposite from the therapist's prediction. For example, if a patient feels sad when he or she is alone, the therapist might ask, "Were you thinking how good it was to have some privacy?"

Once the patient has grasped the concept that his or her automatic thoughts in a situation can powerfully influence feelings, physiology, and behavior, the therapist assigns the patient the first part of the thought record. This means that the patient will record the triggering event, his or her automatic thought, and the subsequent emotion and behavior in the next week. The therapist also instructs the patient to record a measure of the strength of the emotional response and the strength of his or her belief in the automatic thought. This becomes important as new, more rational responses are generated so that the patient and therapist can evaluate the effectiveness of finding a believable response and whether this response helps the patient to feel better. An important caution to the patient is to let him or her know that if he or she feels worse while collecting automatic thoughts throughout the week that he or she should stop, because it is only the first half of the procedure. At this time the patient has not yet been taught to respond to these thoughts, and collecting them can be too painful if the thoughts remain unaddressed.

The therapist's homework for **MR. WHITE** was to complete a thought record. For the first several days, Mr. White wrote down thoughts he had in response to situations with women and when he felt inadequate and embarrassed, such as, "She thinks I'm a jerk. She knows I'm never able to have a decent relationship. Who would want to talk to me?" By the third day, Mr. White skipped his classes and stayed at home to play computer games. His therapist had not instructed him that he could feel worse just by collecting these thoughts and that he should stop doing so if he noticed this pattern.

Many of the current thought record forms employed by cognitive therapists with their patients include printed questions to help patients (and therapists) evaluate thoughts for accuracy. These questions are derived from a particular method of evaluating patients' thoughts called guided discovery. Beck coined this term in 1979 as a way of using the Socratic method to help patients recognize distortions in their thinking. This method uses questions to uncover errors in logic. Beck discovered that this method was much more powerful than simply correcting or pointing out logical errors to patients. Other people in the patient's life have generally pointed out his or her logical and factual errors, and he or she will discount these alternative explanations. The process of gathering evidence and developing alternative explanations is one that the patient must engage in himself or herself to most profoundly affect dysfunctional thinking. The Socratic method of asking questions about thoughts and conclusions becomes a tool a patient learns to use outside of sessions and in the future. Guided discovery uses questioning to help patients look at alternatives to their thinking and behavior. It widens the patient's view of consequences of decisions, behaviors, judgments, and problems. It asks the patient to examine meanings of events and opens up the possibility of alternatives to the rigid thoughts and beliefs he or she has.

In the second part of teaching patients the automatic thought record, patients are taught to evaluate the evidence that supports or refutes the automatic thought and then frame a new thought based on available evidence. The patient is challenged to look for other potential explanations or possible likely outcomes of a situation. The new thought the patient develops is evaluated with respect to its believability and its impact on the patient's mood and behavior. At times, the patient will test a thought by gathering evidence or by changing behavior to see what happens. The therapist must complete the entire thought record with the patient in session to make certain that he or she understands how to do it. Subsequent homework includes asking the patient to collect and respond to thoughts and to bring written thought records to therapy. Homework allows the therapist to further refine the patient's skill in evaluating automatic thoughts. Thought records allow the patient and therapist to begin to recognize common themes and uncover underlying intermediate beliefs and core beliefs, which are then modified. Writing thoughts down is important because it increases the patient's objectivity. Patients learn that thoughts do not necessarily equal facts. In the instance where automatic thoughts are found to be accurate they are identified as problems to be solved, and those problems subsequently are worked on in treatment. An alternative approach to accurate automatic thoughts is to find out what the thought means to the patient—it is often this personal meaning that requires investigation. When changing distorted thinking changes emotions and behaviors, patients decrease those activities that maintain the abnormal emotional state, and improvement in symptoms occurs.

MR. WHITE and his therapist reviewed his second automatic thought record, for which he was assigned to collect thoughts and not respond to them. Mr. White listed several situations when he was in a social setting. On each occasion, he wrote down a thought relating to another person judging him critically. Each time this type of thought occurred, he felt angry and ashamed and left the situation. He rated these situations with respect to the emotional intensity that he felt and the percent belief he had in each thought.

Situation	Automatic thought	Emotion	Rational response	Outcome
In coffee shop, speak to waitress	She thinks I'm stupid. (95%)	Angry (100%)		
		Ashamed (100%)		
Out with friends talking about movie	They are sick of my whining. (90%)	Angry (100%)		
		Ashamed (100%)		

The therapist asked Mr. White several questions about each thought, trying to establish the accuracy of what happened. In the first instance, Mr. White said his evidence for the waitress thinking he was stupid was that she didn't seem to be listening and was distracted when he was talking to her. The therapist asked about the setting in the coffee shop; Mr. White explained it was a crowded Saturday afternoon and the waitress was covering a whole section on her own. The therapist asked if this could have an impact on her attentiveness. Mr. White agreed that it could. In addition, the therapist obtained information from Mr. White that this waitress had been quite friendly to him on other occasions and that this distracted behavior was unusual for her. Finally, the therapist asked Mr. White how likely it was that his remark to the waitress would have caused her to think that he was stupid. Mr. White, after examining the evidence, said he thought this had a less than 30% probability. The therapist reminded Mr. White that the purpose of the thought record was to help him to more accurately assess evidence that might be disregarded by him when he is in a particularly negative mood state, and that he then might be able to arrive at a new way of considering the situation.

The therapist then asked questions about the second situation to evaluate the evidence for Mr. White's thought. Each time the therapist examined the situation, she worked extremely hard to make certain that Mr. White described the situation as carefully as he could and generated as much emotion as possible about the thought in the session. The therapist also worked diligently to find and spend the most time on the thought that made Mr. White feel the worst. In the second instance he said it was that, "Everyone thinks I'm a loser." After they examined each situation thoroughly, Mr. White generated a new thought about the situation and rated his subsequent emotion and belief in the thought. Mr. White began to see that although he had evaluated what had happened in one particular way, there were plausible alternative explanations.

Situation	Automatic thought	Emotion	Rational response	Outcome
In coffee shop, speak to waitress	She thinks I'm stupid. (95%)	Angry (100%) Ashamed (100%)	Lisa is having a bad night. (100%) She seems too distracted to talk. (80%) She's enjoyed talking to me before and came by to say hi. (80%)	Neutral. (100%) I could have stayed and had coffee.
Out with friends talking about movie	They are sick of my whining. (90%) Everyone thinks I'm a loser, because I'm single. (100%)	Angry (100%) Ashamed (100%)	People often ask for and respect my opinions, even though I'm critical of things. (100%) Many of my friends have called me more and said they thought that I was the better person in the relationship. (90%)	Embarrassed about the breakup, but okay with talking about the movie. (90%)

Another tool the therapist can use in helping the patient to modify his or her automatic thoughts is to teach common types of thinking errors. Then patients can sometimes more easily recognize the errors in logic that are commonly made by people and modify their own thoughts. An example is teaching patients the concept of confirmation bias—that is, that people will pay selective attention to experiences that confirm their beliefs. For example, if someone has a negative belief about his or her intelligence, he or she will specifically attend to information confirming his or her stupidity and discount or not notice information that counters this view. Lists of common thinking errors are available in many cognitive therapy texts and include mind reading ("She must think I'm really an idiot"), fortune telling ("If I ask him to go out with me, I'm sure he'll turn me down"), and catastrophizing ("If I don't get the promotion I'll just fall apart"). An example of a list is included in Figure 5-2.

Lists of common thinking errors help the patient to identify biased thinking, and such lists often help the patient to see that biased thinking is a universal experience and not unique to mental illness. Once patients identify errors in their logical thinking they can then begin the process of seeking evidence and formulating rational alternatives.

After obtaining good results in relieving the patient's symptoms by modifying his or her automatic responses, the therapist and patient begin to uncover and evaluate the intermediate beliefs and central themes that govern the patient's behavior and form the foundation of his or her perceptions. Intermediate beliefs are frequently found in the form of rules that people develop to cope with core beliefs and that form expectations about others and themselves in the world. Intermediate beliefs are frequently influenced by culture. For example, children raised by immigrant parents in our culture are often imbued with beliefs about educational achievement and success equating to self-worth. Frequently, patients can test these rules by performing behavioral experiments. Therapists can maximize the curiosity the patient has about whether a rule is actually accurate by formulating the rule as an "If . . ., then . . ." statement. For example, "If I don't have a man, then I will never be happy; If I'm not rich and successful, then I've failed completely." Most dysfunctional intermediate beliefs are absolute and judgmental. The patient experiences these beliefs as true and unalterable. Therapists must skillfully identify and artic-

Although some automatic thoughts are true, many are either untrue or have just a grain of truth. Typical mistakes in thinking include:

1. *All-or-nothing thinking* (also called black-and-white, polarized, or dichotomous thinking): You view a situation in only two categories instead of on a continuum.
   Example: "If I'm not a total success, I'm a failure."

2. *Catastrophizing* (also called fortune telling): You predict the future negatively without considering other, more likely outcomes.
   Example: "I'll be so upset, I won't be able to function at all."

3. *Disqualifying or discounting the positive:* You unreasonably tell yourself that positive experiences, deeds, or qualities do not count.
   Example: "I did that project well, but that doesn't mean I'm competent; I just got lucky."

4. *Emotional reasoning:* You think something must be true because you "feel" (actually believe) it so strongly, ignoring or discounting evidence to the contrary.
   Example: "I know I do a lot of things okay at work, but I still feel like I'm a failure."

5. *Labeling:* You put a fixed, global label on yourself or others without considering that the evidence might more reasonably lead to a less disastrous conclusion.
   Example: "I'm a loser. He's no good."

6. *Magnification/minimization:* When you evaluate yourself, another person, or a situation, you unreasonably magnify the negative and/or minimize the positive.
   Example: "Getting a mediocre evaluation proves how inadequate I am. Getting high marks doesn't mean I'm smart."

7. *Mental filter* (also called selective abstraction): You pay undue attention to one negative detail instead of seeing the whole picture.
   Example: "Because I got one low rating on my evaluation (which also contained several high ratings) it means I'm doing a lousy job."

8. *Mind reading:* You believe you know what others are thinking, failing to consider other, more likely possibilities.
   Example: "He's thinking that I don't know the first thing about this project."

9. *Overgeneralization:* You make a sweeping negative conclusion that goes far beyond the current situation.
   Example: "[Because I felt uncomfortable at the meeting] I don't have what it takes to make friends."

10. *Personalization:* You believe others are behaving negatively because of you, without considering more plausible explanations for their behavior.
    Example: "The repairman was curt to me because I did something wrong."

11. *"Should" and "must" statements* (also called imperatives): You have a precise, fixed idea of how you or others should behave and you overestimate how bad it is that these expectations are not met.
    Example: "It's terrible that I made a mistake. I should always do my best."

12. *Tunnel vision:* You only see the negative aspects of a situation.
    Example: "My son's teacher can't do anything right. He's critical and insensitive and lousy at teaching."

FIGURE 5-2 ■ Thinking Errors. Adapted with permission from Aaron T. Beck, M.D., by Judith S. Beck, Ph.D. Reprinted with permission from *Cognitive Therapy: Basics and Beyond.* New York: The Guilford Press. 1995.

ulate these underlying rules by looking for patterns in the patient's dysfunctional thinking and behavior and then testing hypotheses with the patient. The process of uncovering intermediate beliefs is a wonderful model for the patient of the therapist as a co-investigator. The process teaches patients that the set of personal meanings that they have developed are ideas, not absolutes, and these constructs can be identified and modified.

MS. GREEN and her therapist quickly determined that she had several rules about the need to do things perfectly. One of them was "If I don't do something perfectly, then I'm not trying hard enough." Ms. Green and her therapist examined this rule from a number of new perspectives. First, they named it as a rule she had, and not a fact. Then the therapist asked if Ms. Green thought that everyone should do things perfectly, and if they didn't, whether it was true that they were not trying hard enough. Ms. Green easily thought of a number of times when her friends or family had done their best and did not do a perfect job. The therapist and Ms. Green talked about whether Ms. Green thought that it was reasonable that she should have rules that applied exclusively to her. Ms. Green agreed that this was not reasonable, even if it felt to her that it should be. Finally, the therapist looked with Ms. Green at the advantages and disadvantages of having this rule. Ms. Green made the following chart:

Advantages	Disadvantages
This rule will keep me trying to do my best job.	This rule makes me take longer than I need to on many trivial projects.
	This rule causes me anxiety and stress.
	This rule may not improve my performance.
	This rule may keep me from trying new things.

After evaluating the rule in this way, Ms. Green decided to try and work to relinquish it by doing some of the things she generally tried to do perfectly in an "okay" way to see what happened. She and her therapist planned that she would leave one job undone in the house and evaluate what happened, and that she would cook "average-quality" meals during the week. After a week, Ms. Green reported that no one in her family noticed this change and that she felt less resentful and happier.

Core beliefs are more difficult to modify than automatic thoughts and intermediate beliefs. Changing core beliefs involves a longer period of evidence gathering and gradual reinforcing of new beliefs. Therapists must first introduce the concept of what a core belief is and begin to work on changing core beliefs only when the patient fully understands the cognitive model and is able to modify his or her automatic thoughts. Often the patient's core beliefs are obtained by using the downward arrow technique described by Burns (1989). This is a process by which the therapist uses the patient's automatic thought as a starting point and asks the patient what it would mean if the thought was true rather than looking for confirmatory/disconfirmatory evidence. At each juncture the therapist inquires, "And what would it mean if ____ were true about you?" until the patient arrives at the most basic belief about himself or herself or the situation. This process leads the therapist to understand the more personal meanings a thought might have for the patient. The patient and therapist collaborate and agree on a hypothesis that accounts for the content and formation of the patient's core belief. Patients are taught that these beliefs are ideas that may feel true, but may not actually be true, and that when these beliefs function to process information and alter behavior they appear to be accurate reflections of reality. Core beliefs that most people have are generally positive; those that are negative are frequently activated by particular situations or mood states, and subsequently begin to function to process information and affect behavior. An exception is in personality disorders, when patients have fairly fixed negative core beliefs regarding themselves, other people, or the world. Individuals with personality disorders will often present core beliefs as their automatic thoughts and may need to work on these beliefs earlier in treatment once the lengthy process of establishing the therapeutic relationship is completed (see Chapter 11). Therapists may need to supply new alternative beliefs to patients who have personality disorders, because their developmental experiences and subsequent life may not have provided them with more functional ways to think about themselves or other people.

Each time **MS. GRAY** attempted to do a thought record, her automatic thought was "I'm bad" or "I'm worthless," regardless of the situation. Her emotional response to this thought was generally sadness, although her behavior in response to this varied. She isolated herself, had fights with other people, cut herself, drank, and thought about taking overdoses of medication. Since her therapist was confident about their working relationship and Ms. Gray had largely stopped acting on her impulses to hurt herself, he decided to work on this belief. Her therapist explained that he thought she had a strong enduring idea about herself—that she was bad and worthless. Furthermore, he told her that when things triggered her to have that idea, which happened frequently, she felt horrible and often did things that hurt her or damaged her relationships. Ms. Gray agreed that this happened, but said that her being "bad" wasn't an idea; it was the truth. Her therapist asked her to consider two possibilities, either that she a) was completely bad and worthless or b) believed that she was bad and worthless and therefore acted in ways that were harmful to her and often "proved" her badness. He wondered if Ms. Gray could see that it might be useful and more accurate to think about herself in a different way. She agreed that it would, but saw it as impossible. The therapist asked her what might be an alternative way of thinking of herself. Ms. Gray drew a blank. The therapist asked her what she thought she would tell a friend who believed as she did. Ms. Gray still drew a blank. The therapist asked her if she might consider the belief that she had both bad and good attributes, but sometimes she thought that she was bad and worthless. Ms. Gray said that she could not believe that was accurate, but she was able to see it might be a useful way to think about herself and that it could lead her to behave less destructively. The therapist said it would make sense to determine if there was any evidence that this alternative belief was true. He asked Ms. Gray to make a list of qualities that she thought were good ones for a person to have and qualities that she thought were bad ones. They began by having her observe other people, then adding to and refining the lists. Together they made a list of Ms. Gray's attributes and compared the two lists. She found she had some good attributes and some bad ones. She was instructed to gather evidence over time about the accuracy and inaccuracy of the new belief. This evidence gathering caused her to gradually see herself as less "bad." However, at first, Ms. Gray was easily prone to return to her basic belief of herself as bad and worthless.

A means to help the patient evaluate and modify core beliefs is asking whether the belief can be supported by examining evidence for it over the patient's lifetime. This cognitive continuum can help a patient to formulate a different self-concept. Patients can also weaken the strength of beliefs by defining the meaning of terms; for example, if a patient sees himself or herself as a completely "bad and evil" person, finding historical correlations of individuals he or she would see as "bad and evil" and comparing himself or herself to those individuals can weaken his or her belief.

MS. GRAY and her therapist began to tackle her belief that she was "completely worthless." Her therapist asked her to define a completely worthwhile person and she developed the following list:

1. *Lives on her own.*
2. *Has good relationships.*
3. *Has a good job.*
4. *Doesn't need medicine.*
5. *Everyone likes her.*
6. *Helps other people.*

Before her therapist asked her to look at what a completely worthless person was like, he asked her about the criteria. For example, he asked her if she knew of anyone who lived with her parents or with roommates. And she said, "Sure, Kate." And he asked her, "Do you think of Kate as being less than completely worthwhile?" Ms. Gray said, "No." As they went through the list, she was less and less able to defend many of the criteria of what made someone worthwhile. Eventually, she came up with:

1. *Tries to do her best.*
2. *Is caring toward others.*
3. *Tries to find good and steady employment.*
4. *Helps other people.*

With the definition of worthwhile in hand, Ms. Gray was ready to move on to define worthless. As she did, her standards of worthless did not hold up as rational. Finally, with a good definition she was able to rate from 0% to 100% how she sat on the continuum of worthlessness and found she did not qualify as completely worthless. She was given an assignment to gather evidence supporting or refuting her belief of herself as completely worthless using her new standards.

Once a new belief is generated by the variety of techniques available to the therapist and patient, the patient is instructed to gather evidence that disproves or supports the new belief, as well as evidence that counters or supports the old belief. This period of evidence gathering becomes a long-term assignment.

After several weeks of successfully using automatic thought records to modify his thinking, **MR. WHITE'S** therapist drew his attention to the fact that many of his thoughts seemed to have a central theme—that he was worthless, different, and unlovable. The therapist explained the concept of core beliefs to him and shared her hypothesis with him about how these ideas may have developed in his case. Mr. White agreed that he had always thought this was "how it was," and that he thought it would always be that way. The therapist said that believing these ideas were true might make Mr. White behave as if they were true and that his behavior (withdrawal, avoidance, emotional aloofness) could make other people respond in ways that confirmed his belief. She asked if he would be willing to test his beliefs over time. He agreed to work with her on a continuum. She instructed Mr. White that it was important to look for evidence both for and against the idea that he was totally worthless over his lifetime to see if it was true.

	Evidence for belief, "I'm totally worthless."	
Age	For	Against
0–5		I was just a baby.
		My sisters loved me.
		My grandparents were always happy when I was around.
5–10	Mom yelled at me a lot.	Got good grades.
	Never saw dad.	Played little league.
		Took good care of my dog.
10–15	Mom said I'd never do well with girls.	Mom said she could count on me.
	Didn't have a lot of friends.	Had one good friend in Scouts.
		Won math award.
15–20	Didn't date until college.	Graduated high school.
	Fiancée broke up with me.	Got into good college.
		Worked every summer.
		Lots of people wanted to hire me.
		Had a few good friends.
20–25	Not promoted.	Good uncle to my nieces and nephews.
		Kept job.
		Took care of friend when she was sick.
25–30		
30–35		
35–40		
40–45		

After Mr. White and the therapist completed the continuum he was able to form a new belief about himself: "I've been less successful than I'd like, but I'm still a good person." Mr. White agreed that working to strengthen this belief and increasing skills to help him be more successful socially were good treatment goals. The therapist explained to him that it would be important to rate the strength of his belief in the new belief they had formed in a day-to-day way. He gave Mr. White core belief worksheets (illustrated in Figure 5-3) as useful tools to collect evidence for the core belief over time.

By quantifying the strength of beliefs and emotions throughout treatment, the patient provides the therapist with data about patient progress. More importantly, it gives the patient a different perspective about how much change has occurred and increases the accuracy of his or her predictions. Patients notice that the convictions they hold about themselves vary in intensity from day to day and situation to situation—this can weaken these "absolutes" in their thinking. Finally, by asking the patient to rate on paper the degree of belief that he or she has in particular thoughts and beliefs, the therapist further demonstrates to the patient that these are thoughts and ideas, and not absolute, immutable facts.

Various techniques exist to modify core beliefs, and therapists select what they believe is a good fit for a particular patient. Patients with deprived or traumatic childhood experiences or patients with Axis II disorders often benefit from using role play and imagery to restructure basic ideas they have about themselves. This change procedure needs to be done with thoughtfulness and sensitivity, and therapists benefit from reading and focused practice about the technique (Beck, 1995; Young, Klosko, & Weishaar, 2003).

Core belief work takes longer to accomplish than teaching patients to skillfully change their automatic thoughts. Patients should be assured that it is normal for it to take some time to modify these long believed ideas. It is helpful for the therapist to explain that certain situations may be more prone to activate what remains of a core belief and that the patient may have the opportunity to work again to modify what remains of the belief in the future.

Since symptom relief is a fundamental goal of treatment, the "behavior" in cognitive behavioral therapy is important. One theoretical basis of the treatment procedures of depression in cognitive therapy comes from Lewinsohn's (1974, 1975) theory stating that social learning and positive reinforcement are factors

CORE BELIEF WORKSHEET

Old core belief: I'm inadequate
How much do you believe the old core belief right now? (0–100%) 60%
   *What's the most you've believed it this week? (0–100%) 90%
   *What's the least you've believed it this week? (0–100%) 60%
New belief: I'm adequate in most ways (but I'm only human, too).
How much do you believe the new belief right now? (0–100%) 50%

Evidence that contradicts old core belief and supports new belief	Evidence that supports old core belief with reframe
Did good work on literature paper	Didn't understand econ concept in class, BUT I hadn't read about it and I'll probably understand it later. At worst it's an inadequacy but maybe it's actually her fault for not explaining it well enough.
Asked a question in statistics	
Understand this worksheet	
Got a B on chemistry test	Didn't go to the teaching assistant for help, BUT that doesn't mean I'm inadequate. I was nervous about going because I think I should be able to figure out these things myself and I thought he'd think I was unprepared.
Made decisions about next year	
Arranged to switch phones, bank accounts, insurance, etc.	
Got together all the references I need for econ paper	Got a B on my literature paper, BUT it's an okay grade. If I was really inadequate. I wouldn't even be in college.
Understood most of Chapter 6 in statistics book	
Explained statistics concept to guy down the hall	

*Should situations related to an increase or decrease in the strength of the belief be topics for the agenda?

FIGURE 5-3 ■ Sally's Core Belief Worksheet. Copyright 1993 by Judith S. Beck, Ph. D. Reprinted with permission from *Cognitive Therapy: Basics and Beyond.* New York: The Guilford Press. 1995.

in the initiation and maintenance of depressive states. His theory states that depression occurs in patients because they experience a decrease in overall reinforcement from the external world—due to a decrease in positive reinforcement and/or an increase in negative reinforcement. Depression is conceptualized in this paradigm as a vicious cycle of the patient's gradual withdrawal from positive activity and an exponential loss of positive input. Thus, the therapist needs to work aggressively to increase the depressed patient's engagement in reinforcing activities and social interactions.

Behavioral strategies employed in cognitive therapy are derived from Lewinsohn's (1974, 1975) model of the psychopathology of depression and employed in a flexible way. These strategies are tailored to the specific patient and used as a way to engage the patient, provide symptom relief, and obtain relevant data for the therapeutic process.

The first, activity scheduling and monitoring, can be a powerful tool to use for patients with a variety of disorders. This assignment teaches patients to monitor themselves. The patient is instructed, at minimum, to record his or her activities each hour over a period of days. This recording is done contemporaneously to avoid the distortions that occur because of mood symptoms and faulty memory. The activity schedule can be used flexibly by the clinician and patient to monitor activities (to correct distortions about how a patient thinks he or she is spending time and to rate those activities associated with mastery and pleasure), to schedule pleasant or productive activities (particularly in depressed patients who are doing far fewer of them, or who do not remember what pleasurable events they did in the past), and to identify activities that are associated with strongly positive or negative affect. It provides data to the patient and the therapist about how the patient is functioning. Activity scheduling can be used to plan behavioral assignments and record their results. Activity scheduling removes the need for a depressed patient to decide what to do—he or she is already assigned which activities to try. It gives the patient control over his or her time, recognizes the efforts he or she is making to accomplish things, and records his or her actual accomplishments. It can be a powerful adjunct to use for patients who are in medication management treatment; patients can record side effects, activities, and changes in symptoms. This relatively simple intervention can powerfully link depressive symptoms to a lack of purposeful and positive behavior, setting the stage for problem solving.

> **MR. WHITE** and his therapist agreed that his tendency to isolate himself and his lack of pleasurable activities were problems that he needed to address. He had the belief that "if he wasn't with his girlfriend, he wouldn't have any fun." The therapist and Mr. White made a rating scale of pleasurable events from 1 to 10 that he could use as a benchmark to rate events during the week. She also worked with him to plan three activities to try during the week and asked him to predict how much pleasure he would take in them—they included playing basketball, going to the movies, and seeing a friend for breakfast. He predicted that he would rate each of these activities as a 2 or 3. She asked him to rate these and any other pleasurable activities that he engaged in during the week, to see if he noticed any other fun activities. He predicted that there would be no fun experiences. Mr. White brought his homework to the next session. He was surprised to find that he rated basketball and seeing his friend for breakfast as a 6 and 7, respectively. He rated the movie as a 0, and found five other activities during the week that he felt rated a 5 or 6. He and the therapist analyzed the situation and what it meant about his prior belief. Mr. White said that it was possible for him to enjoy some things more than he had thought, that it improved his mood to do enjoyable things, and that possibly he would not enjoy movies without his girlfriend. This session set the stage for his continuing to engage in more rewarding activities.

Skill deficits are conceptualized in cognitive therapy as potential contributors to depression; for example, if one cannot manage interpersonal relationships, one loses an important opportunity to be reinforced in a positive way. A significant contribution by Beck and others to this paradigm is the idea that, in addition to the decrease in positive reinforcement, the depressed patient further compounds his or her symptoms by the cognitive appraisals and faulty conclusions he or she draws from this lack of positive reinforcement. For example, depressed patients who are doing less and less may conclude that they are helpless. When the therapist helps the patient to change behavior, it provides direct evidence that these cognitive appraisals are incorrect. The patient then has a powerful example of how inaccuracies in his or her thinking led to dysfunctional emotions and behavioral responses. Treatment proceeds in both a cognitive and behavioral way in correcting this problem.

MR. WHITE brought in his first activity schedule. He had not enjoyed any activities in the week he recorded and had spent most of his time alone at home watching television and playing computer games. He was certain that he didn't have the energy to do anything else and that if he tried, he would feel even worse. The therapist asked him how he spent his time on weekends before he got depressed and found out that he enjoyed playing pick-up basketball at the neighborhood recreation center. They contracted for him to go and try this for 20 minutes on Saturday, with the understanding that if he felt worse, he could leave and spend the rest of the day indoors. The therapist carefully obtained his commitment to try this experiment to test out his belief that he would feel worse. The result was that he spent an hour playing basketball, talked to a few acquaintances, felt much better, and agreed to go back the next week. Mr. White and his therapist discussed how his predictions here were inaccurate and likely reflected his negative bias. He agreed to continue to test other negative predictions he made.

Compensatory strategies that patients develop to cope with negative core beliefs also lead to the development of skill deficits and ineffective coping. Cognitive therapists identify and remedy ineffective coping strategies. For example, patients who overuse avoidance and passivity are likely to cope poorly with adversity and will adapt better if they use relationships and problem solving to cope with stressful life events.

When **MS. GRAY** first came to therapy, one of the first problems that she and her therapist tackled was her predisposition to fly into a rage whenever she felt ashamed, humiliated, or upset. This would lead to her cutting herself, having physical fights with people, or acting in ways that were self-destructive to her at work or school. Ms. Gray's therapist asked her why she behaved in ways that were so damaging to her at these times and she said, "I just can't stand how I feel then. It's like I'll explode if I just don't do something." Her therapist identified two problems—first, that she believed that she would be damaged by intense feelings (and this was a belief/idea she had, not necessarily true), and second, that she was vulnerable to excess emotions and needed to find some different ways to manage her intense feelings. Ms. Gray looked puzzled. What became clear to her and to her therapist was that she had never considered, nor been taught, possible ways to help calm herself down when she was upset, but she thought of herself as "bad and evil" whenever she had feelings of anger or sadness.

Behavioral interventions can involve correcting particular skill deficits when the therapist determines that they contribute to the lack of positive reinforcement in the patient's life. The therapist can look at the problem list, the patient's behavior in sessions, and the patient's developmental history for clues as to what skill deficiencies may be present. Parenting, managing emotional states, assertiveness, social skills, time management, and problem solving are all behaviors that are important to assess. Increasing social effectiveness can be a critical component of treatment to reduce depression. If patients have never developed skills that allow them to feel socially competent, teaching them can be extremely helpful to ameliorate the current episode of depression, to subsequently correct distorted thinking, and to prevent future episodes. In Axis II disorders, skill deficits can be especially prominent because of the chronic and pervasive nature of these problems. Many Axis II disorders are associated with early psychologically depriving environments with faulty modeling of healthy psychological skills.

MS. GRAY and her therapist spent several sessions working on helping her to regulate her emotions. They established that her being vulnerable to her emotional state was a problem that led to many behaviors that were destructive to her. She clearly had been raised to think of any emotional display as shameful and weak, and she had never had anyone to teach her to identify emotions or how to deal with her feelings. First her therapist gave her several handouts about what increases a person's vulnerability to emotion so that Ms. Gray could be aware of potentially dangerous situations and do things to reduce her vulnerability. Following that, they began a series of exercises to help Ms. Gray label emotions correctly. The therapist developed a series of coping cards with her that would help her in situations when she felt overwhelmed by her feelings. They returned to this theme and reinforced these skills many times during the initial phase of therapy.

MS. GREEN had an extremely difficult time saying "no" to doing things that she did not want to do. She had never learned how to do this—her own mother had been extremely submissive, and she, in fact, had been taught that it was her duty to be obedient and nice by acceding to the demands of other people. She often felt guilty about trying to avoid things that she didn't want to do without saying directly what it was that she wanted. She would resent it when family members did not predict what it was that she needed, even though she did not ask for it directly. Her therapist pointed out that her lack of direct and assertive communication made it difficult for her to feel satisfied and for other people to be in relationships with her. They discussed the reasons that she learned to communicate in this indirect way. The therapist spent a session with Ms. Green teaching her more assertive ways to communicate, gave her practice exercises, and looked at the thoughts that she had about how other people might relate to her if she could be more direct. Although not every situation had the outcome she desired, Ms. Green was much more satisfied with her relationships and how she spent her time as a result of this intervention.

Finally, cognitive behavioral therapy employs behavioral treatments including graded task assignment and exposure. In graded task assignment, patients develop lists of goals that they have not pursued or problems they have not solved because they have dysfunctional thoughts interfering with these activities. This avoidance can occur in depression because a patient has incorrectly predicted that he or she might feel worse by engaging in an activity. The therapist enlists patients to participate in activities by helping them define a goal, and then they break the situation into more manageable parts. Patients learn to develop a plan to solve a problem by doing easier pieces first. The therapist can also have the patient use cognitive rehearsal to imagine taking these steps toward a goal and identify and troubleshoot roadblocks before he or she begins. The therapist assigns tasks to the patient and evaluates interfering thoughts and beliefs. The patient and therapist evaluate the patient's efforts, revise the plan as needed, and continue to work toward the goal.

Exposure can be useful in anxiety disorders, when a patient has developed an unrealistic fear of a situation. Exposure means helping the patient to endure progressively longer periods of engaging in feared situations—sometimes by first engaging in imaginal exposure. Although more aggressive exposure treatments have the potential to be more rapidly effective, it is often difficult to get the patient to cooperate and engage in activities that are so frightening. Graded exposure allows patients to gradually approach and engage in activities that they have feared. Relaxation techniques are another critically important behavioral tool used by cognitive therapists to combat agitation and to relieve insomnia. Relaxation techniques are used to lower overall tension in generalized anxiety disorder and panic disorder. Specific techniques are required to combat panic disorders and other anxiety disorders; relaxation alone is ineffective. These techniques are detailed in Chapter 10.

Behavioral and cognitive homework assignments are a standard part of each cognitive therapy session. Assignments can include many of the tools discussed in this chapter, including automatic thought records, activity scheduling, behavioral experiments, and reading and reviewing the notes from the previous session. Patients who do homework recover faster and more completely. Homework ensures that the skills learned in therapy generalize and that the patient can employ them in his or her natural environment. The goal of treatment is not to have the patient be a good patient—it is to make certain that the tools of therapy which have been useful to the patient become part of the patient's repertoire of coping skills and responses. The assignments are tailored to the stage of treatment and level of disorder, and can be cognitive and behavioral. Reinforcing what has been learned in therapy is a particular goal of homework; patients review what they learned the previous week, as well as engage in tasks that further their progress. The therapist must be certain to review homework that has been assigned and to troubleshoot any difficulties the patient is having in completing homework. Coping cards—written cards that respond to a patient's typical cognitive distortions or that correct behavioral problems with new learning from therapy—can be effective reminders and reinforce the therapy process.

MR. WHITE recognized with his therapist's help that when he felt more depressed, he used the strategy of decreasing his activity to try and conserve his energy and to not be involved with other people. He realized that this strategy was ineffective and potentially increased his symptoms. He made a card with his therapist to help him to remember this:

When I'm feeling depressed I must:

1. Make certain that I am continuing to do things that I enjoy.
2. Call a friend to go out once per week.
3. Continue to exercise at least three times per week.

MS. GRAY and her therapist made a card for her to use whenever she felt like cutting herself or overdosing. They did this by identifying all the activities that Ms. Gray had done in the past to help her get through difficult times. Ms. Gray agreed to use the card because her goal was to not hurt herself, and agreed to paste copies on her medicine cabinet, phone, computer, and in her purse.

When I feel like I want to cut my body or overdose, I will:

1. *Call Miranda.*
2. *Call the crisis line.*
3. *Call my therapist.*
4. *Go for a walk with the dog.*
5. *Listen to jazz music.*
6. *Take a shower.*
7. *Take a nap.*
8. *Go to a movie.*

If all of these fail, I will go to the ER.

Learning points

- Cognitive therapists use many techniques to help patients to modify automatic thoughts, intermediate beliefs, and core beliefs.
- Behavioral techniques are critical to use to combat inertia and obtain alternative data through exposure.
- Cognitive therapists use techniques flexibly, planning treatment by using the patient conceptualization and stage of therapy.

REFERENCES

Beck, A. T. (1976). *Cognitive therapy and the emotional disorders.* New York: International Universities Press.

Beck, A. T., Rush, A. J., Shaw, B. F., et al. (1979). *Cognitive therapy of depression.* New York: The Guilford Press.

Beck, J. S. (1995). *Cognitive therapy: Basics and beyond.* New York: The Guilford Press.

Burns, D. D. (1989). *The feeling good handbook.* New York: William Morrow.

Dobson, K. S. (Ed). (2001). *Handbook of cognitive-behavioral therapies* (2nd ed.). New York: The Guilford Press.

Greenberger, D., & Padesky, C. (1995). *Mind over mood: Changing how you feel by changing the way you think.* New York: The Guilford Press.

Leahy, R. L. (2003). *Cognitive therapy techniques: A practitioner's guide.* New York: The Guilford Press.

Lewinsohn, P. M. (1974). A behavioral approach to depression. In R. M. Friedman & M. M. Katz (Eds.). *The psychology of depression: Contemporary theory and research.* Washington, D.C.: Winston-Wiley.

Lewinsohn, P. M. (1975). The behavioral study and treatment of depression. In M. Hersen, R. M. Eisler, & P. M. Miller (Eds.). *Progress in behavior modification,* Vol. 1. New York: Academic Press.

Young, J., Klosko, J., & Weishaar, M. E. (2003). *Schema therapy: A practitioner's guide.* New York: The Guilford Press.

Structure of Sessions

LEARNING OBJECTIVES

The reader will be able to:

1. Understand the purpose of the structure of treatment sessions in cognitive behavioral therapy.
2. Learn the particular elements of a typical session.
3. Identify situations that would require that the therapist modify the session structure.

Cognitive behavioral therapy is notorious for being a structured treatment. I use the term notorious because one of the most misunderstood features of the treatment is the structure—leading to the belief that cognitive therapists use a prescribed series of techniques, have a "cookbook formula" for treatment that remains the same for each patient, and are inattentive to the particular needs of individual patients. As with all dysfunctional automatic thoughts, there are some developmental reasons that led to this incorrect belief, and hopefully the evidence in this chapter will correct the misunderstanding.

Cognitive therapy was designed as a psychotherapy that could be empirically tested. Because it was imperative to test its efficacy, manuals for the implementation were designed for research purposes. These manuals made certain that the treatment studied was cognitive therapy and tested different models for particular disorders (i.e., eating disorders) where the method had not been applied. This method of evaluation was unusual compared, for example, to evaluation of psychodynamic psychotherapy, and it has been responsible for some of the misconception that cognitive therapists have a session-by-session script that is applied to each patient. Cognitive therapy does ascribe to the philosophy that it is important to provide patients with as rapid relief as possible from their symptoms and proceeds with an imperative to efficiently plan individualized and unique treatment within and across sessions. Protocols for particular disorders give the therapist a set of useful tools that can help patients at a particular stage in treatment. This hardly implies that the therapist applies the same treatment to each particular patient and ignores the individual. The overarching goals of treatment are to understand the patient's individual experience and symptoms using the cognitive model, to teach the patient to identify and respond to automatic thoughts and core beliefs, and to translate nonspecific problems into practical problems that the therapist and patient can solve. Each patient will have particular stressors that contribute to the development and maintenance of his or her problems and specific coping strategies and beliefs that have produced his or her worldview.

Each individual therapy session in cognitive behavioral therapy has a particular structure. This structure exists for several reasons. It makes certain that any change in symptoms or exacerbation of the disorder is determined at the start of a session so that the therapist has ample time to respond. The structure increases patient comfort with the therapy process because it allows patients to know what to expect in therapy; cognitive therapists do not seek to increase the anxiety of a patient, they attempt to decrease symptoms as rapidly as possible. The structure helps to keep the therapist and patient efficiently focused on solving the patient's problems and furthering his or her goals. It teaches the patient the model for therapy and makes it easier for him or her to learn to use it on his or her own. It provides continuity of learning across sessions and makes certain that the patient understands the concepts that have been discussed within the session. It makes certain that the therapist assigns homework and reviews previous homework. The structure is often most beneficial in the cases of those patients for whom the the complexity of the problem is such that you "don't know where to start."

MS. GRAY'S therapist was completely overwhelmed during the first two sessions. Her problems were serious and causing her enormous distress. She was unable to stay on one topic and constantly referred to her considerable pain. Ms. Gray was offended when the therapist suggested that they set an agenda. When he asked her why, she said that she was certain this meant that he wouldn't listen to how she felt when she had problems and she had so many that they would never solve all of them. The therapist agreed that she had a considerable number of problems. He asked her if any of her prior therapists ever made efforts to solve them one at a time. She said no and that in fact they were sympathetic and let her talk about whatever bothered her most. The therapist pointed out that, despite this, Ms. Gray's problems continued to exist, and perhaps a lack of progress was not because it was hopeless to solve them, but because no one could do much without "a more systematic approach to them." He asked Ms. Gray if she would be willing to try an experiment—that they would work together on whatever problem was bothering her most for a certain time period in the session and then "let her vent," and that they would agree to try to work together to solve her problems in a step-by-step way.

Despite the benefits of the therapy structure, many therapists new to this form of treatment have numerous beliefs about what it will be like to employ the structure within a session—"Patients won't like it; Patients won't get to talk about what's really important unless I just let them talk; It won't be possible for me to respond empathically in a crisis." The evidence indicates otherwise. First, most patients readily accept the structure of treatment when the rationale is presented to them as part of the clinical procedures employed by the therapist. To accomplish this task, the therapist needs to explain to the patient during the first few sessions following assessment what each element of the session is and why it exists. Patients are assigned the task of bringing agenda items to therapy each week—those events they see as particularly bothersome or that they wish to work on—and generally become more efficient at bringing concerns to treatment over time. Collaboratively setting the agenda makes it explicit to the patient that the therapist is interested in what is of concern to him or her to discuss in the session. The structure of the session is subordinate to rule number one: the therapeutic alliance comes first. This means that the therapist must respond to a crisis and do what makes sense even if it means that the planned structure is knowingly ignored for a session. Patients with repeated crises merit special handling.

MS. GREEN came to therapy 15 minutes late. She had just had a minor motor vehicle accident. She was extremely upset. Her pregnant daughter had started spotting the night before and had been placed on bed rest to forestall a threatened miscarriage. The therapist had been planning to review a long homework assignment from the week before, and the plan for the session was to develop a hierarchy of feared situations to start exposure treatment. Because of the circumstances, the therapist told Ms. Green that it made the most sense to table that plan, and instead to talk about her concerns about her daughter and problem solve how best to deal with this situation.

MS. GRAY came to her first several therapy sessions in dramatic crisis. She had multiple suicidal crises (sessions 3, 5, and 7), she was thrown out of her house (session 4), she had physical fights with her boyfriend (sessions 3, 4, and 6), and she spoke with her father and found out that his physical condition was worsening (sessions 7, 8, 9, and 10). Her therapist was constantly concerned for her safety. They were able to agree to work together to help her to avoid harming herself during these repeated crises and solve problems as best they could to decrease the chaos in her life. Ms. Gray talked to her therapist about how she felt that she couldn't live like this anymore. Her therapist agreed that such a chaotic life would feel hard to live with, but that the goal of their work together was to decrease the chaos so that she felt more control. Ms. Gray agreed that the first item on every agenda would be to ascertain her safety, and the second item would be to teach her alternative means to respond to crises. Thereafter, they would work to solve any problem that had surfaced during the week that led her to feeling suicidal.

Sessions typically begin with a review of self-report forms that the patient fills out before the session (i.e., the Beck Depression Inventory [BDI]). These forms serve several useful functions. First, they efficiently gather data for the therapist about the patient's symptoms. Second, they can draw the therapist's attention to new symptoms that must be addressed in that session (i.e., suicidal ideation). Finally, they provide a week-by-week assessment of the progress that the patient is making for both the therapist and the patient, which provides useful feedback about the effectiveness of treatment. The BDI and other useful rating scales are available from The Psychological Corporation at www.Psychcorp.com. If self-report forms are not used, the therapist conducts a brief check of the major symptoms that the patient has—for example, asking the patient to rate his or her mood on a scale from 1 to 10. The therapist then provides a "bridge" from the previous session in order to make certain that the patient understood the salient features and get any additional feedback about the session. The bridge provides for continuity across treatment sessions and reassures the patient that the therapist has maintained an interest in the patient's experience.

The next element of the therapy session is setting the agenda. The therapist does this in consultation with the patient, although the therapist often contributes elements of the agenda. Homework that was done for the current session can either be reviewed as part of the agenda or at a separate time. The agenda combats the patient's inertia and sets the tone for collaboration between patient and therapist. Agenda setting establishes the idea that the therapist and patient work together to relieve the patient's suffering and to understand the origins of his or her symptoms. As therapy proceeds, the patient is more and more responsible to bring items to be discussed in the session. Items are prioritized by the therapist and patient. When faced with too many choices, a collaborative decision occurs in the context of the therapist's clinical judgment about what is reasonable to accomplish (one or two problems is usually plenty), what the overall treatment goal is, what the patient wants to accomplish, and what could have the most impact on the patient's symptoms. It is important for the therapist to choose a problem, or part of a problem, that therapy can reasonably impact in a session. The therapist has the responsibility for maintaining the pace of the session and keeping the focus on the task at hand.

The therapist and patient work in the session to solve the problems on the agenda. It takes skill to efficiently know how much history one needs to begin to work on a particular issue. Beginning therapists are extremely well trained in data collection and will often spend a good deal of therapy time getting a descriptive history about a problem rather than trying to work on the problem with the patient. Working on problems in the session in itself can help the therapist to conceptualize the patient; it can provide information about skill deficits that the patient needs to remedy or inform the therapist that the patient is not implementing solutions because of cognitions that deactivate his or her motivation.

MR. WHITE brought five problems to his second therapy session:

1. Never meeting women.
2. Feeling uncomfortable around people.
3. Not paying bills on time.
4. Staying in bed all day.
5. Hating the way he looked.

Because of the stage of therapy and the therapist's concern about Mr. White's depression, they collaboratively agreed to work on problems three and four. As they set the agenda, the therapist explained that these problems seemed the most urgent and that she thought working with them was most likely to improve his mood. She said that the other problems he presented were good goals to work on in therapy, and that they would pursue them in subsequent weeks.

Periodically during the session the therapist summarizes, or asks the patient to summarize, the important points learned in therapy to reinforce the patient's learning. The therapist tries to teach the patient how the session relates to the patient's short- and long-term goals. Summaries should increase the patient's connection to therapy and his or her motivation to problem solve and do homework. Homework is assigned throughout the session as the therapist thinks of assignments that will further the goals of therapy. Homework that reinforces any change efforts by the patient is optimal. The stage of treatment influences what homework is assigned. Homework is never optional, because patients who do homework recover more rapidly and completely.

Finally, the therapist asks the patient for positive and negative feedback about the session. It is important that the patient writes down the homework and main summaries (in early sessions, or with a depressed patient, it is helpful for the therapist to do the writing) to make certain that learning continues between sessions. A therapy notebook can be a wonderful tool to use for relapse prevention and to ensure better homework compliance.

Learning points

- Cognitive therapy sessions have a particular structure designed to decrease ambiguity, maximize efficiency, and teach patients the tools of treatment.
- Therapists remain empathic to the needs of the patient while setting goals and planning the structure of sessions.
- Summaries and feedback provide critical information to the therapist and facilitate the patient's learning.

REFERENCES

Beck, A. T., Rush, A. J., Shaw, B. F., et al. (1979). *Cognitive therapy of depression*. New York: The Guilford Press

Beck, J. S. (1995). *Cognitive therapy: Basics and beyond*. New York: The Guilford Press.

Dobson, K. S. (Ed.). (2001). *Handbook of cognitive-behavioral therapies* (2nd ed.). New York: The Guilford Press.

Greenberger, D., & Padesky, C. (1995). *Mind over mood: Changing how you feel by changing the way you think*. New York: The Guilford Press

Young, J., Klosko, J., & Weishaar, M. E. (2003). *Schema therapy: A practitioner's guide*. New York: The Guilford Press.

Resistance

LEARNING OBJECTIVES

The reader will be able to:

1. Understand how cognitive behavioral therapists conceptualize resistance.
2. Learn the major techniques for evaluation and intervention with resistant patients.

Cognitive therapists take the practical problems and symptoms that patients bring to treatment and reformulate them to reflect the psychological origins, skill deficits, and reinforcement paradigms that produce or perpetuate these problems and symptoms. Although this sounds straightforward, the execution in therapy is much more complicated. Many reasons exist for resistance—both the patient and the therapist can be responsible for the patient's lack of effective participation. Resistance is defined in cognitive behavioral therapy as the patient's inability to engage in the tasks of therapy. Although there are some differences in the theoretical framework by which resistance is understood by different cognitive theorists, the method of evaluation remains similar. Therapist factors, patient factors, and forces from the patient's external environment are all considered in evaluating why therapy is not proceeding as planned.

A major reason for resistance in cognitive therapy is the failure of the therapist to adequately develop and attend to the therapeutic alliance. Therapist inexperience and therapeutic ambition can contribute to this problem. Patients do not readily engage in therapy if the alliance between therapist and patient is poor. Lack of trust and understanding, as well as empathic failures, can erode patient progress in treatment. Therapists working with patients who have extremely dysfunctional relationships and behaviors can underestimate the difficulty that the patient will have in changing these behaviors, and their interventions will reflect this lack of understanding.

MS. GRAY started her first therapy session on time and was cooperative in answering her therapist's questions. The therapist began the
treatment by talking with Ms. Gray about the behaviors she would need
to change and that there were certain behaviors—particularly overdosing and cutting herself—which the therapist wanted her to stop immediately. The therapist brought out a list of assignments he wanted Ms.
Gray to complete at the start of the second session—including having
her write a brief autobiography. Ms. Gray said little in the session. She
was 20 minutes late to the third session and had done no homework.
The therapist asked Ms. Gray how she expected therapy to work given
her lack of participation. She blurted out impatiently, "That's just it; I
don't expect it to work! It never has and it never will." The therapist
was surprised by the vehemence of her response. He thoughtfully and
quickly said, "You know, you're right. There's no reason for you to
expect therapy to work or to trust me. Maybe we should take a step
back and talk about what you might expect from our relationship."
Ms. Gray reluctantly agreed to more actively participate in therapy until
she could ascertain whether the therapist could be trusted.

Resistance can occur when patients have a history of significant trauma and victimization, with subsequent difficulty developing trusting relationships and initiating the change process.
Patients who have been victimized can believe it is unfair that
they should be required to change, because they have been the
injured party. Therapists can help patients to assume the role of
survivor, rather than victim, and become less symptomatic by
actively coping with problems.

In the initial stages of therapy, **MS. GREEN** was reluctant to be forthcoming about anything, focusing exclusively on the need to find a pill that
would help her to feel better. She frequently derailed discussions to
discuss physical complaints and would constantly apologize for "not getting anywhere." Finally, the therapist talked specifically and empathically

about how difficult it must be for her to have these symptoms and how hard it would be to trust someone and feel so out of control. The therapist said that he knew that Ms. Green would need to gradually build trust in their relationship. Ms. Green was visibly relieved. The therapist asked Ms. Green whether she thought that it could be dangerous to talk about her problems in therapy. Ms. Green said she was concerned that she would be forced to talk about things she didn't want to discuss. The therapist reminded Ms. Green of the structure of the session and pointed out that since she set and agreed to the agenda for the session it was not likely that she could be forced to discuss something she didn't want to discuss. Furthermore, the therapist instructed her specifically to stop the conversation if she felt overwhelmed or threatened and give him feedback if they were moving too quickly. Ms. Green became more relaxed and gradually eased into doing the work of therapy.

A second important type of resistance is procedural resistance. Procedural resistance is defined as the patient not following through with the tasks and limits of therapy. Procedural resistance can stem from difficulties with the therapist or the patient. Therapists must adequately explain, and patients must, in turn, understand the rationale for the framework and assigned tasks in treatment. The patient must understand the particulars and must be able to do what the therapist is asking; that is, he or she must have the skill to perform the task. Therapists can determine if the patient can complete a task by having the patient complete a small part of the homework in the session. Therapists need to make certain that assigned homework makes sense to the patient. The therapist must identify and resolve obstacles, both practical and psychological, that can interfere with the completion of tasks.

MR. WHITE'S therapist was pressed for time at the end of a session. She gave him a thought record and as he was leaving, said, "Try and jot down a few of the negative thoughts you have this week." Mr. White became overwhelmed when he tried to do the assignment, felt more depressed, and did not complete the task.

Resistance to the structure and limits of therapy can also be a reflection of the patient's typical interpersonal functioning. The therapist can evaluate this by determining if the resistance fits with the patient's past patterns. Patients who are dependent, who are impulsive, or who have significant need for autonomy are frequently experienced by therapists as resistant. Approaching the resistance in a matter-of-fact and nonjudgmental way is often the course to a successful outcome.

MR. WHITE brought his therapy homework in every second or third session, often without completing the entire assignment. The therapist had a few early problems with incompletely explaining the homework but thereafter was diligent at making certain that Mr. White clearly understood the assignment and how it would benefit him. The therapist tried to understand the problem Mr. White was having with the homework by reviewing his conceptualization and history. At his next visit, she put the problem Mr. White was having with homework completion on the agenda. She asked Mr. White what his thoughts were when he was doing homework assignments. Mr. White told her that he felt that the assignments were "busy work" and that he "shouldn't be made to do menial work." The therapist was surprised and asked Mr. White whether he had had similar thoughts about assignments in other settings—like at school or work. Mr. White said that he always felt that "bogus" assignments and needing to "suck up" to other people made him angry. He felt that he should not be requested to perform in this way to get along in the world. Mr. White's therapist used this opportunity to address this belief that he had and that there might be advantages and disadvantages of continuing to behave in accordance with this idea, particularly with regard to work and school assignments. The therapist suggested that they use the therapy homework to explore this problem. She worked with Mr. White to generate a list of advantages and disadvantages of doing work proposed by his therapist. Mr. White then acknowledged that there could be an advantage in participating in the homework. The therapist asked Mr. White if he had considered that he was choosing whether or not to do the homework—in effect, not being "made" to do anything. Mr. White agreed to try an experiment to evaluate how he would actually feel if he completed homework assignments and to identify thoughts that he had while doing these assignments and evaluate them for accuracy. In addition to increasing his capacity to participate in therapy homework, Mr. White uncovered a number of beliefs that he had about how intolerable it would be to be controlled by other people. These beliefs were a substantial hindrance to his work and personal life, and he was at least able to note them as ideas that he had, rather than facts that needed to govern every one of his choices.

When avoiding emotion, some patients can appear to be resistant. This avoidance generally stems from ideas and beliefs that emotions are dangerous or weak. Emotions can feel threatening to many patients, particularly when they have catastrophic beliefs about experiencing feelings ("I'll never stop being sad if I let myself; People don't respect you if you let your emotions show"). Surmounting resistance in these situations involves testing the validity of these beliefs.

The patient can appear to be resistant when the therapist has incorrectly or incompletely conceptualized the patient's history and presenting problems. The therapist could simply be "barking up the wrong tree." Sharing the conceptualization with the patient frequently increases the patient's sense of being understood and clarifies areas that are not well explained by the therapist's view of the patient. The therapist may not have all the necessary data that he or she needs to help the patient.

In the early months of therapy, **MR. WHITE'S** therapist conceptualized his problem as relating to fears of criticism and beliefs about being controlled by other people that had been activated by the breakup of his relationship. Despite multiple efforts to increase his social contacts, Mr. White continued to avoid being with most people. The therapist reviewed the conceptualization she had with Mr. White, asking him if he agreed with her understanding of his development and the contributions of the events of the recent past. He said he did, but that he saw the problem as his extreme anxiety in most social settings and his belief that he was likely to do something to incur the ridicule of others. He said that his fears of criticism were so severe that he could focus on nothing except his anxiety and that he wanted to avoid and escape all such situations. She got further information about his reactions to social encounters and found that he met the criteria for social anxiety disorder and had developed this problem in early adolescence. After reconceptualizing Mr. White's difficulties, Mr. White's therapist began to work differently with his avoidance and therapy proceeded more smoothly.

Cognitive behavioral therapists sometimes consider resistance from the standpoint of reinforcement. It is easy to forget that immediate positive consequences always have a stronger impact than delayed negative ones. Often what appears to the therapist as resistance is the result of contingencies that reinforce the patient's maladaptive behavior. These contingencies can be internal (psychological) or external (from the patient's system or social network). Family and the social framework of the patient can provide the patient with powerful incentives to continue his or her current behavior. Changing the reinforcement paradigm, helping the patient use cognitive strategies to set goals, and increasing the patient's tolerance of delaying gratification can often help with resistance stemming from lack of reinforcement.

When **MS. GREEN** had episodes of severe anxiety, her sister gave her one of her alprazolam tablets. Ms. Green felt relief from this and had developed a strong learned response to the situation: that when she felt her worst, alprazolam would fix the problem. She was extremely reluctant to stop doing this, and in fact was not certain that she could tolerate the feelings of anxiety that she had any other way. Ms. Green's primary care physician had been reluctant to prescribe benzodiazepines for her and told her that she "could get hooked." Ms. Green's therapist explained to her that when someone is having a panic attack, they easily develop a powerful attachment to medication that relieves their distress because of the terrifying nature of the symptoms. The therapist asked Ms. Green if there had been times when she had tolerated the panic symptoms because her sister was not available. This indeed had been the case. After educating Ms. Green about panic disorder and the dis-advantages of taking benzodiazepines in response to an increase in symptoms, Ms. Green agreed to try and not use medications to deal with her symptoms, and if it became intolerable, to work with her therapist to find alternative ways of managing her anxiety. The therapist, in turn, agreed to provide Ms. Green with a number of strategies she could try to use to manage her anxiety in urgent situations until they were able to get the disorder under control.

Cognitive behavioral therapists also try to consider whether the patient has a high level of reactance. Reactance is an individual's effort to restore a sense of personal control whenever he or she is threatened with a loss of autonomy. Describing the current set of problem behaviors to the patient and having him or her predict the outcome if he or she continues to engage in these dysfunctional behaviors can, over time, facilitate making the choice to change. If resistance is a characteristic in all of the patient's relationships, the therapist can manage it by using paradoxical interventions, nondirective assignments, and by making certain that the patient is truly engaged in collaborating with the therapist in the work of guided discovery. Rational emotive behavior therapy (REBT) theorists have addressed the issue of resistance in therapy and advise therapists to adopt an accepting attitude toward the patient; to continually encourage change; to point out to the patient the consequences of not changing; and to be flexible, innovative, and experimental in the approach to the patient. Many of the techniques developed by Miller and Rollnick (2002) in their work with motivational interviewing are helpful in working with the patient with a high level of reactance.

Faced with **MR. WHITE'S** extreme reluctance to try new behaviors, the therapist asked him to answer the rhetorical question that he posed, namely, "What's the use of trying?" She seriously entertained the question with him and asked him to generate a list of advantages and disadvantages of trying new behaviors. She emphasized that it was always his choice to try new things and that he would always control the speed of the change process. He made the decision to try the next behavioral experiment and he kept the advantage/disadvantage analysis to use at other times when he felt "stuck" when contemplating a new task.

Linehan (1993), in her writing about treating borderline personality with dialectical behavior therapy (DBT), describes another important source of overcoming resistance. She notes that patients with borderline disorders need to be validated simultaneously with the demand for change in therapy. DBT describes the borderline personality patient's experience of the therapist's directives to change as being similar to the invalidating environment that he or she experienced in childhood, and therefore it promotes resistance. For patients to whom the structure of cognitive therapy feels invalidating, the therapist can tailor interventions to include more clarification, empathic restatement, and self-directed homework to help the patient experience a greater sense of collaboration and move toward change.

MS. GRAY developed another therapeutic impasse when her therapist began to work to help her to more effectively communicate her needs to other people. Despite agreeing that this was a problem that often led her to be furious and to impulsively provoke the other person or hurt herself, she refused to productively engage in role play with her therapist or to practice any skills outside of the session. The therapist reviewed his plan: he had carefully broken the task into small and gradually more challenging parts; he had an agreement with the patient regarding the need to change this behavior; and he had explained the rationale for the change procedures clearly. He confronted Ms. Gray with her lack of follow through and she said, "You just do not understand. This is too difficult for me to do. I'll never be able to manage it." The therapist discussed the situation with a supervisor and the next week told Ms. Gray that he understood that this process was a frightening and difficult one, fraught with situations that Ms. Gray had spent her life avoiding. He told her that he was aware that his asking her to try this was terrifying for her, but that he believed she was capable of trying difficult things. She was then able to do the first role play with him.

Validation can take the form of the therapist assuming that the patient is attempting to problem solve with less functional behaviors. The therapist must understand the value of these behaviors to the patient and communicate this understanding to the patient. Patients often face difficult dilemmas, along with real losses that will occur as a result of the changes and decisions that they make in therapy. Patients may accurately appraise consequences to other people resulting from their changing in therapy. Acknowledging this is extremely helpful in producing behavioral change.

Many cognitive therapists (Beck, 1995; Leahy, 2001; Young, Klosko, & Weishaar, 2003) have noted that resistant patients need to change core beliefs in order to change problematic behavior. When patients have core beliefs that are extremely painful (e.g., "I am worthless; I am completely defective"), they will engage in strategies to avoid or compensate for these and to keep themselves from being exposed to these beliefs. If therapists do not address the underlying belief, they will have a difficult time obtaining any meaningful change in the problematic strategies that the patient uses. Core beliefs about change can be a problem (e.g., "Change is dangerous"), and the consistent activation of core beliefs can cause the patient to consistently interpret benign events and interpersonal interactions in a negative way. Patients who have had multiple episodes of illness or who have had unsuccessful treatment can have beliefs about change that are formed by actual experience that therapists must counter for treatment to proceed effectively.

Although **MS. GREEN** had agreed that her constant worry was a problem, she was extremely reluctant to do anything to decrease the amount of time that she kept doing it. She was given a number of behavioral strategies to reduce the amount of time she spent worrying, and she knew from her therapist that her worry increased the panic symptoms that she had. She only half-heartedly engaged in any homework about decreasing worry. Ms. Green's therapist decided to tackle this by asking Ms. Green what she was afraid would happen if she stopped worrying, and what it would mean about her if she worried less about her family. From this exploration the therapist found that Ms. Green believed that she would be overwhelmed by fears and feelings if she did not worry and that if she didn't worry about her family it would mean that she didn't care about them. These testable beliefs became a focus for therapy, and after Ms. Green had modified them, she was able to more actively participate in decreasing her worry.

When resistance is due to core beliefs about efficacy, the patient who does not believe he or she has the ability to complete an assignment will not attempt it. Cognitive therapists use many strategies to modify core beliefs, including historical tests of the core belief over time, behavioral experiments, and evaluating and understanding the origins of these beliefs (see Chapter 5).

Behavior change can only occur if the patient has skills present to engage in new behavior. If patients cannot do what is being asked of them, they will not do it. Therapists must assess the skill level of the patient via historical assessment, role play, and focused practice. If the skill is not present, the therapist must teach the patient the new behavior before change can occur. Often, an individual has had repeated episodes of failure in skill acquisition because of his or her temperament, and reframing of past experiences in light of this understanding can be helpful in the acquisition of new skills.

Therapists must also help patients who have poor self-management skills (e.g., time management, stress reduction, behavioral reminders) to acquire these to make it possible for the patient to adequately participate in treatment. Patients who lack the opportunity to do homework will not do homework.

MR. WHITE was chronically disorganized about his therapy assignments and about many things involving his personal life. For example, he frequently forgot to write down phone messages and call people back; he would neglect getting his hair cut; and he did not plan time to go grocery shopping. The therapist asked him how he kept track of his personal time, and he had no mechanism for this. He agreed to experiment with using a calendar to plan and schedule such personal needs. His careful attention to this skill produced positive results. He explained to the therapist that he had never considered that these issues were important enough to plan and that he never learned this in his family life.

Learning points

- Cognitive behavioral therapists define resistance as the failure to engage in the tasks of therapy. It can stem from the behavior of the therapist, the temperament and skills of the patient, and the patient's beliefs about change.
- Accurate case conceptualization and careful attention to the therapeutic relationship are critical tasks for therapists to avoid resistance in their patients.

REFERENCES

Beck, J. S. (1995). *Cognitive therapy: Basics and beyond.* New York: The Guilford Press.

Leahy, R. (2001). *Overcoming resistance in cognitive therapy.* New York: The Guilford Press.

Linehan, M. (1993). *Cognitive-behavioral treatment of borderline personality disorder.* New York: The Guilford Press.

Miller, W., & Rollnick, S. (2002). *Motivational interviewing* (2nd ed.). New York: The Guilford Press.

Young, J., Klosko, J., & Weishaar, M. E. (2003). *Schema therapy: A practitioner's guide.* New York: The Guilford Press.

Termination

LEARNING OBJECTIVES

The reader will be able to:

1. Use several tools to help patients plan for termination.
2. Understand the conceptualization of termination in cognitive therapy.
3. Employ strategies for relapse prevention in patients.

Termination in cognitive therapy proceeds as a logical extension of the therapy itself. Cognitive therapists begin the process of therapy with the explicit goal of making the patient his or her own therapist. This goal is accomplished by teaching the patient the model of therapy, sharing with the patient the therapist's conceptualization of the patient's problem and refining it over time, helping the patient employ the tools of therapy outside of sessions, and predicting and planning for setbacks and relapses. Because the model is essentially one that focuses on learning new skills to solve problems and to evaluate perceptions and thinking for accuracy, termination also takes into account the principle that newly learned skills will need to be reinforced and reviewed on a gradually diminishing schedule. This is commonly done with a series of "booster sessions," which are scheduled with gradually decreasing frequency from the time of termination.

Booster sessions have a structure that is similar to every other cognitive therapy session, except that the intervals between sessions involve longer periods, and the goal of the session is to work on any particular problems the patient has had in employing the skills learned in treatment and for the therapist to assess the patient for relapse. Patients are given homework between booster sessions and are instructed to contact the therapist should symptoms arise between sessions.

Preparing a patient in cognitive therapy for termination is consistent with the model as well. The therapist and patient begin the process by eliciting what automatic thoughts the patient has about the process of termination. The therapist and patient work together using Socratic questioning, and patients evaluate these thoughts for accuracy.

MS. GREEN was visibly upset by her therapist's suggestion that she would soon be capable of coming to sessions less frequently. The therapist quickly asked her, "What just went through your mind?" Ms. Green said, "I'm worried I'll just fall apart again." The therapist first normalized Ms. Green's anxiety about termination and discussed with her how common it is for patients to be worried about becoming symptomatic. He then carefully led her through an examination of evidence for and against her "falling apart" that included specific examples of her independently using the tools of therapy outside the sessions. She was much less anxious, and her reformulated thought was, "It's normal to be worried about ending therapy, but I've learned a lot about dealing with my problems on my own."

Another main feature of preparing a patient for termination involves predicting problems that the patient might have in the future and beginning the process of generating potential solutions to those problems. This process allows the patient to evaluate the capacity he or she would have to employ the skills of treatment in difficult situations in the future, as well as to troubleshoot situations that are likely to be triggers for the patient's problems.

MS. GREEN brought a homework assignment back to her therapist, listing potential problems she might face in the future. The most upsetting one was that her daughter would have complications with her delivery and the baby would have health problems. Ms. Green and her therapist identified this situation as one that might increase her worry and anxiety, and then the therapist assigned her the task of generating a list of the things that she had learned to do to combat such symptoms. Ms. Green immediately listed five things that she could do, including relaxation exercises, exercise, dysfunctional thought recording, scheduling worry, and distraction. She also surprised the therapist by including the novel idea that she would limit the information seeking she would do on the Internet, as it tended to increase her anxiety. The therapist was visibly delighted, and it strengthened Ms. Green's belief that she could cope. The therapist also added that Ms. Green could seek consultation if she was having difficulty employing the tools of treatment or if they were not helping her with her symptoms.

Many patients benefit from using the tools of relapse prevention in preparing for termination. Those patients with chronic difficulties with addiction, eating disorders, or other habit disorders can benefit by the identification of triggers and strategies to help reinforce the avoidance of these triggers. Planning strategies and behaviors to employ during an occurrence of relapse is critical. Patients benefit from distinguishing slips from relapses. This identification means that if a patient engages in a problem behavior once, it does not mean that he or she will necessarily return to having the full-blown disorder. Therefore, just because patients have labeled a slip "hopeless," they cannot give themselves permission to further engage in the behavior. Patients are encouraged to look at brief returns to prior behaviors as evidence that they have improved and to use them as experiments where they can collect data to reinforce their plan for recovery. Patients can generate scenarios that will evoke problematic behavior and then, through imagery, successfully generate more adaptive responses to these situations, which can give the therapist and patient more confidence that the patient can cope with termination.

MS. GRAY worked hard during therapy to stop using alcohol during times when she felt anxious or unable to tolerate her emotional state. As she and her therapist started to talk about decreasing the frequency of her sessions, she found that she was more prone to increasing the frequency of her alcohol use. She and her therapist noted this as a problem and identified the trigger that led to her drinking. The therapist had Ms. Gray imagine another triggering situation. Ms. Gray did so, and then she

> worked with the therapist to generate alternative solutions to drinking and to reevaluate the permission-giving beliefs she engaged in when she slipped. Ms. Gray talked with the therapist about her anxiety about decreasing sessions, and they worked to identify what supports would help her with the transition to being less involved in therapy.

Homework assignments can help the patient prepare for termination, as the previous case examples illustrate. Patients can generate coping cards, review their therapy notes to see what progress has been made and what tools have been acquired, and engage in "self-therapy sessions." Self-therapy sessions are useful for patients throughout treatment at times when they will miss a session. The process involves the patient using the structure of the therapy session to solve a particular problem on his or her own, including assigning homework and generating feedback. The patient will benefit most from this process if he or she keeps notes about what happened—again, similar to the process of therapy. If the therapist uses self-therapy sessions throughout treatment (e.g., during vacations) the patient will approach termination with more confidence.

Finally, the therapist and patient have a genuine relationship to acknowledge and relinquish as a part of termination. Every good therapist will develop his or her own way of discussing this with a patient—again, tailoring this discussion to the needs of the particular patient and in the same collaborative way that characterizes the treatment.

As **MR. WHITE** was approaching his last few sessions, he mentioned to the therapist that he was feeling sad about stopping therapy. Mr. White's therapist acknowledged that this feeling was common, and that she, too, often had mixed feelings about termination—sad that the relationship was ending, happy that the patient had done well, and proud of the patient's accomplishments. Mr. White told the therapist that he felt she was "always in his corner" and that the support of the therapist had made it possible for him to learn new ways of thinking about himself.

Cognitive therapy fundamentally underscores the importance of the therapeutic alliance. Termination must include an acknowledgment of the powerful relationship that exists between therapist and patient.

Learning points

- Cognitive therapy anticipates termination from the start of treatment, with the philosophy that the patient will learn the tools of therapy and use them to continue to work on problems in the future.
- The anticipation of termination is approached with problem solving and thought records.
- Booster sessions are a planned part of treatment to make certain that gains made in therapy continue in the future.

REFERENCES

Beck, J. S. (1995). *Cognitive therapy: Basics and beyond.* New York: The Guilford Press.

Leahy, R. (1996). *Cognitive therapy: Basic principles and applications.* Northvale, NJ: Jason Aronson, Inc.

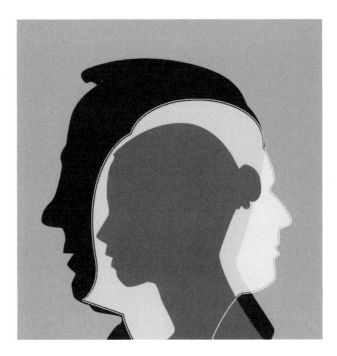

Cognitive Models of Psychological Disorders

Affective Disorders

LEARNING OBJECTIVES

The reader will be able to:

1. State the cognitive model for depression.
2. Understand the relationship between dysfunctional thoughts and behaviors and the symptoms of affective disorders.
3. Be aware of interventions that can reduce symptoms in depression and mania.
4. Learn a cognitive approach to deal with suicidal ideation.

Cognitive therapy for depression is a well-established and effective treatment, with substantial literature supporting its use. Cognitive therapy is superior to the condition of no treatment and equal to other forms of psychotherapy and pharmacological interventions in mild, moderate, and severe depression. Recent studies indicate that cognitive therapy is superior to pharmacological management of depression in the prevention of relapse and recurrence, with cognitive therapy as effective as keeping patients on medication in the prevention of relapse after therapy withdrawal (Hollon, Derubeis, Shelton, et al., 2005). Combining cognitive therapy with medication increases the efficacy of treatment. In a large study of chronically depressed patients, combining a form of cognitive therapy (CBASP) and medication was significantly more effective than either modality given as a single treatment (Keller, Mc Cullough, Klein, et al., 2005). In addition, unlike in the treatment of anxiety, combining cognitive therapy and medication for depression does not seem to diminish the efficacy of either treatment.

The model cognitive therapists have for the development of depression is a stress–diathesis model. A variety of sources predispose people to the development of depression. Genetics and biological predisposition obviously impact an individual's risk for affective disturbance. Multiple psychological risk factors from early development are regarded as risks for the future development of affective disorder. These risk factors can include parental depression—in addition to genetic loading, children will model the cognitive style of their parents, and therefore make similar faulty inferences about negative life experiences that would place them at risk for future depression. Parents who are abusive or neglectful can engender negative expectations and beliefs about the self. Lack of caring and warmth, or critical and hostile parents, also predispose a child to future depression. Early significant losses are also a risk. When an individual has the predisposition to evaluate neutral events as negative, has negative core beliefs, or uses rumination and worry to manage emotions when a stressful life event occurs, he or she is more vulnerable to develop depression in the face of negative life events. Each depressed person is seen to have a personal set of rules and often unarticulated biases that integrate his or her perceptions and life experience. When these are activated, they replace more logical ways of organizing and evaluating information.

> **MR. WHITE** described himself to his therapist as "someone who always expects the worst." When his therapist asked him what he meant by that, he told her that he was always on guard so that he wouldn't be disappointed. He felt that this made life easier than "getting his hopes up." He also thought that he would be weak if he allowed himself to be caught off guard by disappointment. Mr. White, as a result of these beliefs, was constantly sensitive in all of his relationships to anything that could be a sign of potential rejection. He saw this sensitivity as a means of self-protection, and the end result was that he shared little about himself in relationships. He did not understand that his behavior stifled his intimate relationships and that his tendency to focus on negative events and circumstances, as well as to blame himself for not avoiding negative events, increased his vulnerability to depression.

When a person with risk factors for depression is faced with a stressful circumstance (and these circumstances can be stressful for anyone, or stressful to this particular person because of his or her background and experience), he or she can begin to evaluate information in a skewed and negative way. This negative method of information processing creates distorted views about the self, the future, and other people. As mentioned in previous chapters, the "cognitive triad" of negative views about the self, the world, and the future eventually represents most of the person's thinking (Beck, Rush, Shaw, & Emery, 1979). The depressed patient sees himself or herself as bad, worthless, defective, or damaging. He or she evaluates all of his or her negative experiences based on his or her own personal defects. The world is seen as completely depriving and negative, placing unrelenting demands and impossible problems in his or her way. There are no positive experiences to look toward, and relationships are experienced as depriving or certain to be lost. He or she sees the future as unrelentingly bleak and hopeless. Once activated, his or her core beliefs regarding failure, loss, or worthlessness will function as information processors for all incoming data. The patient discounts any evidence that would alter his or her negative mood state. This skewed evaluation leads to sadness, a change in behavior toward others, and a decrease in engagement in previously valued activities. The individual withdraws from pleasurable events and productive behavior. He or she becomes isolated from others, or alternatively sees himself or herself as incapable and depends excessively on the input of others. This isolation and lack of productive and pleasurable activity leads to fewer positive and fulfilling experiences and less evidence to refute negative thoughts. When the patient has a lack of pleasurable activity, he or she will be lethargic and develop a decrease in the capacity to notice pleasurable feelings. Hopelessness, low mood, and suicidal thinking are further reactions to this barrage of painful, negative information.

MR. WHITE became extremely isolated following the breakup with his girlfriend. He felt irritable and sad and had recurrent thoughts that he was "worthless and no good with women." As he ran into friends on campus, he would be sensitive about any friend talking with him about his prior relationship, and think, "He thinks I'm a loser." He began to avoid people because it felt "safer than being laughed at." At first, he did not accept invitations and eventually did not answer his phone. Mr. White felt less and less energetic as time went on. He would say, "This is it" when asked about a social or personal life. He told his therapist, "I've always been like this—I shouldn't have expected life to be any different for me."

Complementing the original hypotheses about depression by Beck et al. (1979), attribution theory, proposed and studied by Abramson, Metalsky, and Alloy (1989) went further to explain the cognitive vulnerability to depression. It states that those individuals more prone to depression tend to attribute negative life events to stable, internal (personality-based) causes. The theory further states that individuals prone to depression believe that negative life events will have long-term deleterious consequences. This attributional style leads to multiple errors in logic; it causes people to blame themselves for events over which they have no control and to engage in fewer potentially positive activities because of the possibility of incurring negative consequences (and feeling worse). This lack of purposeful, positive activity produces more depression and is interpreted frequently by the person as evidence that he or she is incompetent and ineffectual.

The structure of cognitive therapy in itself combats the learning and memory dysfunction associated with depression. Depressed patients do not have normal cognitive function. Their thought processes are slower and their concentration and memory decreased. The methodical and precise session-to-session format of therapy allows the patient to more easily participate in treatment and to learn the important tools to combat symptoms. Treatment of depression begins by educating the patient about the nature of depression and about the therapy itself. The therapist actively assesses the patient's mood state and suicidal and hopeless thinking at every session and aggressively targets pessimism and suicidal thinking and behavior. The therapeutic relationship and the active and collaborative stance of the therapist is a potent tool in combating the hopelessness of depressed patients. Because the therapist maintains a high level of activity, the inertia and passivity of the depressed patient cannot hijack therapy. Additionally, the therapist can actively coach and cheerlead the patient to behave differently, thereby combating the behavioral withdrawal so characteristic of depression. Patients who are depressed cannot always talk it out and need behavior change to demonstrate that the thoughts and beliefs that they have are distorted. Early in treatment, patients are taught how to monitor themselves, set goals, and list the problems to be solved in therapy. Goal setting can quickly target hopelessness by better defining the patient's problems. The therapist can directly confront hopelessness about change if more circumscribed problems are available to solve, providing evidence to the patient that change is possible.

> **MR. WHITE** set goals in an early treatment session to respond to his friends' phone calls and go out once per week. He set this goal reluctantly, and it was in response to the therapist asking him, "What would you be doing differently if you were doing better and not so depressed?" Mr. White was convinced that if he spent any time outside his apartment he would be "in for more rejection and ridicule" and then feel worse. His therapist asked him if he would be willing to test this out by going to the movies with a trusted friend. Mr. White agreed to go and had a pleasant time.

Behavioral techniques are used early in the treatment of depression. The cornerstone of early stage cognitive therapy treatment for depression is to increase a patient's constructive and goal-directed activities. An exception to this is in the case of extremely hopeless or suicidal patients, when these cognitions must be the therapist's initial priority. Activity scheduling, mastery and pleasure ratings, and graded task assignment are powerful tools to combat depression. The increase in positive, purposeful activity breaks a vicious cycle of withdrawal and is an effective treatment for anhedonia and low energy (physical activity improves mood). Patients have a significant increase in their sense of control, and as they gradually increase the pleasurable activities in their life, they have an increase in mood, self-efficacy, and satisfaction. An increase in activity may increase social interactions and improve mood by increasing interpersonal contact and support. Often, depressed patients are reluctant to try to increase social or physical activity because they are afraid that they will feel worse as a result. Using the idea of experimenting with small increments of activity and collecting data is a way to examine evidence about these dysfunctional beliefs. Therapists also use cognitive and behavioral techniques to help normalize sleep and eating and to assist the patient to resume better self-care. This also improves mood and functioning. Behavioral techniques are important in managing depression in the depressed patient who has a significant amount of anxiety associated with the affective disorder. Increasing exposure to feared situations, followed by identifying and restructuring maladaptive cognitions associated with anxiety, assists these patients. Relaxation exercises are particularly helpful for those patients who have more generalized anxiety and worry associated with their depression, particularly if the therapist teaches the techniques in session and schedules focused practice with the patient.

While working with **MR. WHITE,** his therapist determined that he had significant and lifelong anxiety when in nearly all social situations. A main reason for his lack of relationships was that he had an idea that he would do or say something foolish that would expose him to ridicule. He endured social events by using a variety of safety behaviors (see Chapter 10), including drinking and smoking marijuana. Substance abuse played a vital part in his forming new relationships with women, and overusing substances often led him to be incapable of sustaining an erection, furthering his sense of inferiority and humiliation. Mr. White agreed to go to a group targeting his social anxiety in addition to his individual therapy after his therapist pointed out that Mr. White's chance of reaching the goal of a normal social life and relationships and his goal of feeling less depressed would be severely compromised by his social anxiety.

Once a patient has an increase in activity and better self-care, the therapist works to teach the patient how to monitor and record thoughts and how to evaluate thoughts for accuracy. When behavior change has occurred first, it helps to demonstrate to the patient that his or her depressed conclusions are incorrect. The patient learns to develop rational alternatives to the distorted thinking that he or she is believing and uses behavioral experiments, when needed, to test hypotheses and predictions. The patient's dysfunctional beliefs must be uncovered and changed in order for the therapy to have an enduring effect. Looking for these beliefs and linking them to the patient's developmental and interpersonal history helps the patient to have a context for the development of the disorder. Therapists use methods such as evidence gathering, advantage/disadvantage analysis, developing and testing more rational alternatives, and coping cards to help the patient correct the inflexible and rigid ideas that he or she has that would put him or her at risk for future episodes of depression. At times the therapist will work with the patient to modify dysfunctional beliefs about other people that would lead to chronically unsatisfying interpersonal relationships. Therapists also evaluate and target skill deficits, for example, lack of assertiveness, that would be potential risk factors for future depressive episodes. Therapy is individually planned based on the patient conceptualization and symptoms.

MR. WHITE and his therapist worked together to understand the origin of his negative beliefs about himself and other people. She reminded him that he had grown up virtually an only child and that his older sisters often seemed to have "all the answers," doing things far more easily than he did. He grew up with the idea that "if I tried hard enough my mother (or someone) would love me." His birthmark and his size accentuated his chronic sense of "not being good enough." He began to be teased by other children in middle school and at that time began to feel physically panicked when he was in groups of children. He learned his anxiety would decrease if he was alone so he stayed that way as much as he could. He missed school for multiple somatic symptoms and felt like "it wasn't worth going anyway." He compensated for his feeling inferior and less socially adept by chronically criticizing others and developing self-righteous ideas about his values and way of life, despite feeling lonely and isolated. His self-focused attention, when he anxiously scanned for the criticism of others, made him less attentive to another person's point of view. His social anxiety contributed to his negative beliefs about himself and left him vulnerable to depression.

The later stages of therapy for depression involve summarizing the new learning of therapy and consolidating gains. Patients review therapy notes, evaluate the steps taken to reach goals, and predict future pitfalls and problems with the therapist. The therapist reviews with the patient what possible responses he or she could have if future problems did occur and what strategies and skills the patient could employ to avoid future depression. Termination involves the therapist eliciting and responding to patients' thoughts about ending treatment and scheduling booster sessions to make certain that the patient maintains gains met in treatment.

An important concern in patients with mood disorders is the risk of suicide. Assessing the patient with these disorders for thoughts about death must be routine. Cognitive therapists contend with hopelessness and suicidal thinking in an aggressive and targeted fashion. The therapist must manage his or her own anxiety and use a well-planned series of questions and interventions to manage the patient. The therapeutic alliance is most fundamental to treatment in this situation—the therapist must impart hope and a sense that the patient's life is important. Obviously, patients at imminent risk for self-harm are managed by making certain that they are in a protected environment until the crisis passes. The therapist chooses this option after carefully assessing risk factors and empathically acknowledging the pain the patient is experiencing. Using rating scales at the beginning of each visit can quickly access information about the patient's level of hopelessness and suicidal thinking. It is not the sole means of assessment; therapists maintain a high level of awareness about the risk for hopelessness and suicidal thinking in depression and inquire about these at each visit. Therapists target hopelessness, the patient's reasons to live, and reasons and motivations for suicide with suicidal patients by evaluating the accuracy of the thoughts and the consequences of suicidal behavior. Patients construct lists of reasons to be hopeful or reasons to stay alive with the therapist and as homework. Suicidal ideation is explored in detail, with a particular emphasis on identifying what problem the patient is attempting to solve with suicide. The therapist and patient attempt to find alternative, acceptable, and less costly solutions to the problem. The therapist must actively help the patient solve problems in this situation, intervening whenever the patient is unable to generate solutions on his or her own. It is important for the therapist to counter thoughts that the patient has that contribute to his or her wish to die. Thoughts that focus on self-hate, thoughts that endorse suicide as a means of relief, or thoughts that suicide will have particular interpersonal effects contribute to the suicidal patient's intent. Therapists can remind patients of the time-limited nature of crisis situations. Patients who are suicidal are frequently individuals who have had multiple crises and survived—therapists can help the patient by reviewing other times when the patient thought he or she would not be able to cope and used alternative strategies to suicide to manage the situation.

Hopelessness can be confronted by making vague problems specific. Directly asking the patient what he or she is hopeless about and generating a specific problem list allows the therapist to aggressively address each problem. The patient may have thoughts that interfere with solving the problem or have no resources to cope with significant problems. Therapists can help by evaluating automatic thoughts for evidence and by providing assistance when the patient needs ancillary supports. The therapist can help the patient to generate a list of things that the patient can anticipate more hopefully, as such information will have likely been ignored by the patient.

A strategy for the therapist in working with suicidal patients is to use a time line with the patient to have him or her look at what he or she would miss in the future if he or she were dead. Patients often need the therapist to help them reality test what it would mean to die and to have the possibility of no future. The therapist asks the patient what would make life worth living and teaches the patient how to begin the process of putting these reasons for living in place in his or her life. The therapist can ask the patient to answer rhetorical questions that lead him or her to suicidal thinking, for example, if the patient asks, "What is the use of trying to change?" The therapist can ask the patient to list all the reasons it is worth making the attempt to change. Breaking problems down into more manageable parts and exploring with the patient what he or she sees as hopeless about each part can generate hope. Coping cards with specific safety plans and reasons for living can serve as potent between-session reminders for patients. Increasing social supports can also be critical.

MS. GRAY and her therapist agreed early in treatment that her repeated overdosing on medication was a behavior that had significant negative consequences. She agreed to evaluate the advantages and disadvantages of continuing to overdose and developed the following list:

Advantages of Overdosing:

1. People pay attention to me.
2. I go to sleep and forget.
3. It distracts me from my problems.

Disadvantages of Overdosing:

1. People think of me as a mental patient who can't handle things.
2. I could die.
3. My problems are still there when I wake up.
4. I hate throwing up.
5. The dog needs to get put in a kennel.

As a result of generating these lists, Ms. Gray made the decision to try and stop overdosing when she felt hopeless and unable to cope. She made a more extensive coping card with her therapist, which they called a crisis card, to help her at these times.

Crisis Card

When I feel hopeless and like I want to take all my pills, I will take the following steps:

Breathe deeply and focus on my breathing for 5 minutes.

Call three friends—Steve, Nancy, and Irene—until I successfully reach one of them to talk. If they offer help I must accept the offer.

Go for a walk in the park no matter what the weather. If it is after 9 P.M., use the treadmill for 30 minutes while listening to salsa music on my headphones.

Call Dr. Black. If I get the answering service, I must wait for a return call.

Play ball with Buster for 10 minutes.

Call the suicide crisis line.

I agree to preserve my health and safety by going to the emergency room before I overdose if these strategies do not decrease my urge to harm myself.

BIPOLAR DISORDER

Bipolar disorder is effectively treated with adjunctive cognitive therapy. Patients have more robust medication adherence and better recognition of episodes with the addition of cognitive therapy. Bipolar patients who are less well controlled on medications have a high risk of suicide and psychiatric hospitalization, as well as comorbid psychiatric disorders. Several studies (Lam, Jones, Hayward, & Bright, 1999) point to the effectiveness of adjunctive cognitive behavioral therapy in reducing the frequency and intensity of episodic mood disturbance. Because bipolar disorder has many psychological symptoms and sequalae, psychotherapy is helpful even for the patient with bipolar disorder who has reasonable mood control on medication. Monica Basco and A. John Rush (1996) described the adaptation of cognitive therapy for this disorder. The treatment protocol presupposes that the patient has first been stabilized on medication because of the substantial disturbance of thought process that occurs in mania. Treatment has five major components, including educating the patient about the disorder, maximizing lifestyle and medication adherence, developing an awareness of early onset of symptoms and triggers for the disorder, using cognitive behavioral strategies to control symptoms, and dealing with the psychological consequences of contending with a chronic mental illness. Treatment of bipolar disorder with cognitive therapy also takes into account the substantial psychosocial consequences and developmental delays that can be associated with this illness. The original treatment was designed as a manual-based protocol continued over 12 months; therapists can tailor this to the needs of a particular patient.

Therapists using cognitive therapy for bipolar disorder establish the therapeutic alliance and teach the model and concepts of therapy to the patient during periods of stability. The alliance is critical and based on a collaborative and active therapeutic relationship that emphasizes understanding this particular patient's experience of bipolar disorder. The therapist assumes an attitude of helping the patient to cope by enhancing and amplifying already existing coping strategies and including significant others and family members. An explicit and significant goal of treatment is to maximize medication and positive lifestyle changes by problem solving the practical and psychological obstacles to medication adherence and by understanding and correcting dysfunctional beliefs about the meaning of the illness to the patient. The lifestyle issues that are critical to bipolar patients include taking medication, sleeping regularly and sufficiently, managing negative automatic thoughts, monitoring mood, managing stress and stimulation, and discontinuing substance use. Treatment begins by engaging the patient as an active participant using whatever techniques are necessary to establish the idea that psychological treatment and medication management could be life-saving and life-enhancing. Education about bipolar disorder comes first—about the nature of the illness and its symptoms, the nature of the pharmacological treatments used to counter the illness, and the lifestyle issues that increase the likelihood of episodes. Patients are taught to be better observers of symptoms that warrant medication by doing a detailed analysis of the symptoms that typically occur for them in each mood state and then putting into place a consistent method of self-monitoring for these symptoms. Patients are also taught techniques to monitor medication adherence and to evaluate and contend with life stresses. Thoughts that interfere with medication adherence are especially targeted. Side effects of medication are aggressively managed with the goal of having the patient take medication as accurately as possible. The therapist and patient actively take responsibility to make medication use as easy and tolerable as possible. Patients are taught standard cognitive therapy techniques to help cope with depressive cognitions. Manic behaviors are targeted as symptoms that are desirable to keep in check, and generally this occurs by doing a more realistic advantage/disadvantage analysis of becoming manic. Psychosocial difficulties and legitimate grieving associated with having the diagnosis are the final focus of therapy and can include remediation of skill deficits that have resulted from developmental delays, the psychological effects of having unpredictable moods and a chronic psychiatric illness, and anxiety about possible new episodes. When it is necessary the therapist works to confront denial of the illness or its severity. Life stressors associated with episodes of illness are identified (e.g., sleep disturbance, interpersonal stressors) and plans put into place to contend with these as much as possible.

Learning points

- Cognitive therapy has developed specific interventions that are helpful to patients with major depression and bipolar disorder.
- Suicidal patients benefit from the therapist particularly focusing on hopelessness and rigid cognitions they develop about themselves, the world, and the future.
- Behavioral activation is an essential part of cognitive therapy for severe depression.

REFERENCES

Abramson, L. Y., Metalsky, G. I., & Alloy, L. (1989). Hopelessness depression: A theory-based subtype of depression. *Psychological Review, 96,* 358–372.

Basco, M. R., & Rush, A. J. (1996). *Cognitive-behavioral therapy for bipolar disorder.* New York: The Guilford Press.

Beck, A. T., Rush, A. J., Shaw, B. F., et al. (1979). *Cognitive therapy of depression.* New York: The Guilford Press.

Beck, J. S. (1995). *Cognitive therapy: Basics and beyond.* New York: The Guilford Press.

Dobson, K. S. (Ed.). (2001). *Handbook of cognitive-behavioral therapies* (2nd ed.). New York: The Guilford Press.

Ellis, T. E., & Newman, C. F. (1996). *Choosing to live: How to defeat suicide through cognitive therapy.* Oakland, CA: New Harbinger Publications, Inc.

Greenberger, D., & Padesky, C. (1995). *Mind over mood: Changing how you feel by changing the way you think.* New York: The Guilford Press.

Hollon, S. D., Derubeis, R. J., Shelton, R.C., et al. (2005). Prevention of relapse following cognitive therapy vs. medications in moderate to severe depression. *Archives of General Psychiatry 62:* 417–422.

Keller, M. B., Mc Cullough, J.P., Klein, D.N., et al. (2000).The acute treatment of chronic major depression: A comparison of nefazodone, psychotherapy and their combination. *New England Journal of Medicine 342:* 1462–1470.

Lam, D. H., Jones, S. H., Hayward, P., et al. (1999). *Cognitive therapy for bipolar disorder: A therapist's guide to concepts, methods and practice.* Chichester:* John Wiley & Sons.

Linehan, M. (1993). *Cognitive-behavioral treatment of borderline personality disorder.* New York: The Guilford Press.

McCullough, J. P. (1999). *Treatment for chronic depression: Cognitive behavioral analysis system of psychotherapy.* New York: The Guilford Press.

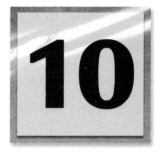

Anxiety Disorders

LEARNING OBJECTIVES

The reader will be able to:

1. State the cognitive model for panic disorder, social phobia, and generalized anxiety disorder.
2. Learn techniques useful in the management of these disorders.
3. Understand the principles of exposure and cognitive restructuring in anxiety disorders.

The cognitive model for all anxiety disorders begins with the observation that anxious patients tend to overestimate the probability of the occurrence of negative events and overestimate the costs of such events to them (probability and severity distortions, respectively). Patients with anxiety err in their estimation of the capacity to cope with adversity and the resources that they have to cope with it. This underestimation leads them to draw incorrect conclusions about the actual risk of a situation. Patients with anxiety disorder believe that they are threatened by danger and react and behave accordingly. Examples of anxiety disorders that have effectively responded to cognitive therapy approaches when empirically tested include panic disorder and social phobia. The purpose of this chapter is to review models for these particular disorders and briefly detail the forms of treatment available.

PANIC DISORDER

In 1985, Beck proposed a model for anxiety that included the idea that anxious patients overestimate risks. Similar to the cognitive model for depression, it begins with the premise that actual events are not what generate the patient's symptoms, but that the patient's interpretation of events leads to anxiety. Biological systems are activated when an individual misinterprets internal or external events, resulting in the characteristic physiologic concomitants of anxiety, including automatic reactivity ("fight, flight, or defend"), inhibition of learning and current behaviors (freeze), and scanning for danger in the environment.

David Barlow (1988), in his work with exposure-based treatments, and David Clark (1986, 1988), further elucidated the model for panic and added to the explanation of the disorder by observing that patients with panic catastrophically misinterpret normal body sensations. When individuals misinterpret normal body sensations as dangerous, the biological cascade that occurs can lead to further anxiety and subsequent panic. Patients with anxiety disorders were also identified as individuals who had a lower threshold for arousal. The patient with panic appraises danger from internal and external triggers, has apprehension and the belief in impending catastrophe, then experiences further anxiety symptoms, overbreathing, a catastrophic misinterpretation of physiological symptoms, and subsequent panic. Once attacks occur, avoidance of the physiologic symptoms and situations where panic occurs perpetuate the catastrophic misinterpretation and lead to further disability. Additionally, individuals become much more hypervigilant for physical symptoms that they interpret as evidence of potential physiological disaster. Important types of avoidance behaviors identified by the cognitive model are behaviors called safety behaviors (Salkovskis, 1996). Safety behaviors are defined as actual avoidance of situations or symptoms; escape once symptoms begin; and thoughts or behaviors that patients employ when symptoms begin, which the patient believes are the only reason catastrophe has not occurred. The concept of safety behaviors helps to explain why patients with panic continue to believe they are in danger even though they have dramatic evidence that no actual catastrophe has occurred. For example, consider an individual who has palpitations and who believes that he or she is having a heart attack. He or she goes to the emergency room and is told that there is no problem with his or her heart but that he or she has anxiety. It would logically follow that if he or she knew that he or she did not have a heart problem, he or she would believe in the future that these palpitations were not dangerous. In individuals with panic, the belief about danger persists because they feel that they have thwarted the heart attack in some fashion either by getting to the hospital in time, by stopping activity just in time, or getting lucky, and that the calamity is still close at hand. Cognitive therapy for panic has been empirically tested and is highly effective; it is as effective as pharmacological management and more enduring after treatment is withdrawn at preventing relapse (Barlow, Gorman, Shear, & Woods, 2000).

MS. GREEN carried a few of her sister's alprazolam tablets with her whenever she was going alone to an unfamiliar place. If she noticed her heart beating she would think, "If I get nervous, I can take a pill and it will calm me down so nothing bad happens to me." The thought of the pill by itself would frequently be sufficient to calm her down. She would further believe that the reason she was able to safely go to unfamiliar places was that she would have alprazolam with her.

Panic disorder patients learn to avoid having anxiety symptoms by using distraction when they develop feared physical sensations. Panic disorder patients frequently develop a variety of behaviors that prevent them from focusing on the symptoms and sensations that they have when confronted with an anxiety-provoking situation that they cannot avoid. Avoidance can also take the form of avoidance of situations and places that are associated with panic, and the patient eventually develops agoraphobic avoidance. Patients with agoraphobic avoidance are more difficult to treat and take longer to recover.

Treatment of panic attacks fundamentally involves reducing the overestimation of disastrous events and correcting the catastrophic misinterpretations about body sensations that patients develop. A number of techniques are employed to help patients correct these errors in their thinking. The first part of treatment involves educating the patient about panic and anxiety and teaching the cognitive model for these disorders. This process is similar to cognitive therapy for other conditions. Patients are taught that the reason for their symptoms is because they have misinterpreted a normal physiologic phenomenon. The analogy of a car alarm triggered in the absence of an actual burglar can help explain to patients why they can have such an outpouring of symptoms even though there is no danger. The therapist can explain that there is a vicious cycle of normal physiologic responses that occurs when the patient interprets a situation as dangerous. Once the patient is taught the theory of panic as conceptualized in cognitive therapy and about the normal physiological processes that occur in humans during a dangerous situation, a number of procedures are available to test if this theory is applicable to his or her particular set of symptoms.

MS. GREEN'S therapist spent a fair amount of time in her session explaining how a normal fear response in humans was to quickly appraise the risk that exists and the resources the person has to deal with the risk. Furthermore, he told her that the problem in anxious people was that they often made errors by overestimating the degree of risk that exists in a situation and underestimating the resources that they have available to deal with it. Further, he explained the natural mechanisms of fight or flight that occur in animals (and humans) and that when Ms. Green considered a situation to be dangerous (like believing she was having a heart attack), her body was likely to respond by increasing levels of chemicals that would increase her physiological response to a frightening situation. Unfortunately, this would further produce physical symptoms that would convince her that she was in physical peril from a heart problem and increase her psychological symptoms.

Treatment of panic disorder then proceeds by obtaining a detailed description of the person's panic attack along with his or her cognitions during the attack. This is most effectively accomplished by asking the patient to describe the most recent or most severe episode. The therapist asks detailed questions about emotions, thoughts, and images, and physical symptoms and behaviors before, during, and after the attack. The patient is also asked to rate the severity of the symptoms during the attack on a scale of severity (0 to 100%). Patients are taught to keep records of their anxiety symptoms, including where they occurred, what particular physiological symptoms they noticed, how severe those were, and what thoughts and beliefs came about at that time. Additionally, patients record their behavioral response to the panic. The most critical item to include in the history is a careful discussion of what thoughts and beliefs occur with body sensations, as it is the patient's interpretation of these sensations that is the cornerstone of what triggers the panic episode.

Treatment planning requires a history of the patient's patterns of avoidance. This history must include a description of any use of distraction or safety behaviors. The clinician needs to ask specifically about situations the patient avoids, physical sensations that he or she avoids, things that he or she does for self-protection, and things he or she does in anxiety-provoking situations that neutralize the thoughts and symptoms he or she has. This detail helps the therapist develop behavioral experiments that most efficiently expose the patient to feared situations.

The therapist must also obtain a developmental history to form an accurate conceptualization, which, in addition to the history of current symptoms and thoughts, gives clues to the therapist regarding particular beliefs the patient has developed that could put him or her at higher risk for panic attacks and reoccurrence. The cognitive style of anxious patients—with the predisposition to cognitive distortions regarding the probability of negative events and severity of the consequences of these events—is important to address with Socratic questioning and a careful examination of the evidence. Anxious patients often underestimate coping resources available to them when faced with threats. Typical beliefs anxious patients have can consist of beliefs about control (it's terrible to lose control), about physical symptoms (people often suddenly die), or about perfectionism (if I make a mistake or look foolish then it's a disaster). Beliefs about worry are often important in the conceptualization of anxious patients—"Good mothers worry about their children; If I don't worry things will fall apart"—and need to be corrected to prevent further difficulties in the future. History taking in any patient with anxiety requires understanding and removing chemical triggers of anxiety, as well as gathering information about medical conditions which either predispose the patient to certain physical sensations or have led him or her to be concerned about being in physical danger.

 MS. GREEN had significant concerns about having a heart attack. She was constantly vigilant about her heartbeat and focused on every perceived irregularity in her pulse or breathing. She talked with her therapist about her concern about having a heart problem. He discovered her family history of cardiovascular illness was significant. A number of her uncles had had early heart attacks and her four grandparents had died in their fifties from heart attack or stroke. Ms. Green firmly believed that if "they all had gotten to the hospital earlier, it would have saved them." She also believed that her "nerves" could make it more likely that she would have a heart attack and had read several studies on the Internet that linked anxiety to cardiovascular disease. This meant that every time she felt anxious, she had the thought that her heart was in danger.

Ms. Green's therapist worked over several weeks to broaden Ms. Green's understanding of the causes of cardiovascular disease, as well as to help her to have a more realistic view of how much control she could expect to have over her cardiac function. One belief they specifically discussed was, "If I got too upset, then I could have a heart attack." Ms. Green's therapist asked her to assess how much she believed that emotional upset could cause her to have a myocardial infarction and die, given that she had just been told by her physician that her heart was healthy. Ms. Green and the therapist worked together to discover how her hypervigilance about physical sensations increased her awareness of these sensations and she subsequently drew the conclusion that a catastrophe was imminent.

The next part of treatment in panic patients is called panic induction. This technique involves inducing the sensations that the patient gets during panic attacks in the therapy session and having the patient evaluate the meaning of those sensations at the time the sensations occur. The rationale for panic induction is that it causes the patient to experience panic symptoms and, while having the symptoms, accurately determine the danger while in the presence of another observer. Panic induction can function as a tool to help to identify the patient's catastrophic misinterpretations, because the aroused and anxious state he or she is in at the time of an actual panic attack is often a barrier to identifying the thoughts and personal meanings the patient has about this event. Panic induction helps the patient to eliminate the belief that the symptoms are dangerous, because it dramatically illustrates the lack of real danger in the physical sensations the patient is having. It demonstrates to the patient that he or she can produce the same symptoms that occur during panic, at any time, without dangerous consequences. It functions as an exposure treatment as well, desensitizing the patient to the panic symptoms. Panic induction teaches the patient that his or her symptoms are normal variations of physical experience. Particular techniques used to induce symptoms and expose the patient to feared sensations include hyperventilating, inducing dizziness (spinning), increasing the patient's heart rate via exercise, and so forth. The goal of panic induction is to demonstrate that it is the catastrophic thinking that the patient has during the physical sensation that leads to panic and not the physical sensation itself. The patient understands that evaluating the catastrophic thoughts for accuracy when he or she has physical symptoms is the solution to decreasing the panic attacks.

Cognitive therapists further help patients with panic disorders to change catastrophic misinterpretation during panic by having them fill out dysfunctional thought records and test conclusions outside of sessions. Thought recording is particularly useful as a tool to pinpoint the patient's avoidance behaviors. Patients and therapists can design particular behavioral experiments to challenge idiosyncratic thinking and avoidance behaviors. For example, patients can be instructed to exercise outside the session and notice that an increased heart rate or an increased breathing rate does not signify danger or the certainty of a panic episode.

A particularly difficult homework assignment for **MS. GREEN** was to exercise at the gym for 5-minute intervals on the treadmill and then focus her attention on her pounding heart, while noticing all the thoughts that came to her mind and working to re-evaluate these thoughts. She was not able to accomplish this assignment at first, but after two sessions during which her therapist had her run in place in the office to increase her symptoms and discuss her thinking at the time, she was able to do it.

Although exposure to the physical sensations associated with panic is a treatment goal, early in treatment a patient may need to manage symptoms. Panic symptoms can be particularly disabling during the period when the alliance is being developed, and the patient is learning about the illness and the rationale for treatment procedures. When necessary, patients can be taught to decrease disabling symptoms of panic attacks. Tools that can help include distraction, controlled breathing to decrease hyperventilation, and focusing on external stimuli during anxious moments. The patient must be instructed that this is a temporary stopgap measure, because the physical symptoms that he or she has are not actually dangerous. Using these techniques helps the patient to function better day to day until exposure and cognitive restructuring decreases the panic symptoms. Patients can also use therapy notes and thought records to help them between sessions. Relaxation techniques, at first practiced when the patient is not acutely anxious, can be extremely helpful. Relaxation and other habits that promote better psychological health and well being (i.e., regular sleep, good nutrition, and exercise) can lower the patient's propensity to have panic attacks.

Exposure is a critical element of the cognitive therapy treatment of all anxiety disorders, particularly when avoidance has become disabling or is maintaining the problem. The therapist begins by explaining what exposure is and the evidence for the effectiveness of exposure as a treatment. Reminding the patient of the therapy goals he or she has set is often necessary because the concept of actually confronting the feared situation seems so threatening. Patients are more motivated to participate in exposure treatment when they understand the rationale and effectiveness of the treatment. A reluctant patient can develop a list of the advantages and disadvantages of enduring exposure with the therapist and become more engaged. Exposure, on the surface, seems counter to reasonable behavior—if something terrifies you, the most fundamental instinct is to avoid it at all costs. A more gradual method of exposure begins with developing hierarchies of feared solutions with the patient, doing imaginal exposure, and then employing gradual controlled amounts of actual exposure to feared situations. More intense and longer exposure to the feared situation is more rapidly effective for anxiety, but many times it is difficult for patients to agree to engage in it. Actual exposure requires a degree of therapist support that is often difficult to obtain. The patient participating in exposure treatment is taught to write down what he or she predicts will happen and how awful he or she predicts he or she will feel when faced with a feared situation. After facing the feared situation, he or she is instructed to evaluate the outcome. Almost invariably the fear the patient has is much greater than what actually happens when exposed to the situation. This makes subsequent trials easier. As exposure treatment proceeds, the therapist must identify any subtle clues that the patient is avoiding sensations or distracting himself or herself. For example, someone who is afraid of public speaking may have the catastrophic belief that he or she may fall from fainting because he or she will be terribly anxious as he or she speaks, and therefore will hold on tightly to the podium. If this subtle avoidance is not noted during exposure and confronted by the therapist, the patient will not refute this hypothesis and it will negate the effects of exposure.

MS. GREEN and her therapist made a list of all the situations she had avoided since developing panic attacks. At first the list was brief, basically involving her not taking public transportation. Her therapist asked her if she was willing to go alone into stores or shopping malls and she said, "No." She and her husband also had a fight in the past week because she made him park the car and come into the drugstore with her, rather than to have him wait double-parked when she went in to pick up a prescription. She said to her therapist, "I just feel better if someone else is there." She and her therapist returned to the list and included places that she avoided being by herself and it was far longer, including:

Taking the bus.
Taking the train.
Riding in a car with someone driving other than my husband and
    daughters.
Going to the store (any type).
Walking at the mall.
Going to church.

Ms. Green and her therapist began by choosing which of these situations seemed the most dangerous and uncomfortable, which one seemed the least, and they put the items in ascending order of discomfort. This list allowed them to choose going to church alone as what she was going to try first. The therapist worked with Ms. Green to break down the steps involved in going to church alone so Ms. Green could accomplish this goal in stages.

Treating individuals with panic disorder and other anxiety disorders with cognitive therapy involves obtaining the patient's agreement to slowly taper benzodiazepine medication used for anxiety. Adequate exposure to feared sensations cannot occur when benzodiazepine antianxiety medication is prescribed. Additionally, the idea of having medications available that will quickly take away symptoms functions as a safety behavior. Benzodiazepines also interfere with a patient's anticipatory anxiety, so the patient may not have dysfunctional thoughts when anticipating feared events that need to be disconfirmed during therapy. Patients need to identify and challenge beliefs they have about continuing medication, slowly taper their medication, and then engage in further exposure treatment.

MS. GREEN had a long-standing problem with using medications to help her to feel better at times of stress and discomfort. This pattern included overusing codeine for a period of years for headache and backache, trying a number of antianxiety medications prescribed without success, and taking alprazolam "borrowed" from her sister. She attributed the lack of success that she had had in using medications for relief to the fact that "doctors don't listen to me and don't really know what they are doing." Ms. Green was initially certain that there would be a pill to correct her symptoms because they were "physical and not psychological." Furthermore, she was convinced that having her sister's alprazolam was the only thing that kept her from "disaster" during several anxious moments. Ms. Green's therapist needed to spend several sessions discussing and evaluating these beliefs and educating Ms. Green about the actual effects of benzodiazepines before Ms. Green was willing to accept a "trial period without medication" because she believed "I'll just fall apart without medicine." Besides educating her about using benzodiazepines, her therapist also reminded her about several difficult periods of her life when she had no medication and managed "without falling apart." He and Ms. Green navigated the potential impasse over using medication by considering it as a "choice she could always make" if therapy did not help her to feel less anxious.

The final important element of working with individuals with panic involves working with images. Many individuals with anxiety disorders have a substantial number of mental pictures involving danger and feared situations that act as triggers for the symptoms that they have. Identifying these mental pictures and responding to them rationally can be helpful in preventing panic and anxiety. Individuals can respond to thoughts and images by actually substituting images of coping effectively for the pictures of disaster that they have. Catastrophic thinking about the image can be corrected in treatment. Repeated exposure to catastrophic images can decrease the emotional response patients have to them.

Whenever MS. GREEN thought about her pregnant daughter, she became anxious. She could not articulate any thoughts that she had about her daughter, but when asked if she any "mental pictures" when she thought about her daughter, she had a strong reaction. Ms. Green had consistent images of her daughter having a miscarriage or dying in childbirth and would be horrified by these images.

She felt like she couldn't cope if this catastrophe occurred, and she worried that having such horrible images could "jinx" her daughter's pregnancy. Ms. Green's therapist helped her through a series of Socratic questions to understand that thoughts and images are not harmful and cannot make things happen. In addition, he worked to help Ms. Green mentally manipulate the image—including seeing herself coping with a less then positive outcome and seeing her daughter's pregnancy have a positive outcome. Ms. Green found that changing the image increased her comfort with her own thinking. She stopped trying to avoid thinking about her daughter's pregnancy and the images became less powerful.

SOCIAL PHOBIA

The cognitive model for social phobia and the treatment protocols that have been established and tested are based on the conceptualization that individuals with social phobia have a basic belief that they are defective and inadequate. Further, patients with social phobia are worried that the discovery of this inadequacy in a social setting (speaking, eating, writing are often the feared activities) will lead to ridicule and negative evaluation by others. Heimberg and Becker (2002) have been instrumental in developing and testing this model, particularly in group treatments, and have demonstrated that cognitive therapy produces results equal to that of pharmacotherapy for social phobia. Therapeutic gains are maintained over a longer period after therapy is withdrawn than when patients are treated with medication. The three major components of cognitive therapy treatment for social phobia are education about the disorder, exposure to feared situations, and cognitive restructuring. The latter two components occur both in session (particularly when patients are in a group) and during homework assignments outside of therapy. Patients are coached in focused practice during therapy sessions about exposure to feared social situations before actual exposure. Coaching allows the therapist to assess for and remedy any social skills deficits and to identify and instruct the patient to not use safety behaviors in practice outside the session. Patients develop a hierarchy of feared social situations and gradually initiate encounters with other people and situations that they would have previously avoided. The patient is asked to

rate the distress he or she has anticipating facing the feared circumstance and subsequently is asked to rate how distressing the
actual experience was.

Exposure procedures allow the patient to identify and evaluate cognitive distortions about failing or being ridiculed in social
situations. The therapist must assess the patient for and confront
negative self-evaluation after behavioral experiments. It is imperative to help the patient avoid paying selective attention to
negative feedback. As the patient corrects his or her cognitive distortions and practices skills in social settings, his or her performance improves. Group treatment with other individuals who
have the same disorder is frequently extremely helpful; the other
group members become credible sources of information to the patient and empathize with his or her experience. In a group, exposure can initially occur in a safer environment and practice can be
more controlled.

 MR. WHITE joined a group to help him deal with his social anxiety. He
developed a list of things that made him anxious, which included:

- Calling a woman for a date.
- Going out with friends when there are new people there.
- Going to parties.
- Meeting new people at school or work.
- Asking for help in a store or the library.
- Going to the gym when it is crowded.

Mr. White placed these situations in ascending order of how fearful he
was about them and was assigned to work on asking for help in the
store, the least uncomfortable situation. He role-played a situation in a
store in group with another group member. First, the group member
played a cooperative clerk, and then, a less interested one. The group
helped Mr. White correct incorrect ideas he had about his performance
during the role play ("I'm sure I looked nervous"), and the therapist
made a videotape of the role play to show him in order to correct his
misconceptions. Finally, Mr. White was given a homework assignment
to go to three different stores in the next week, ask for help at each one,
and report about his experience to the group.

A basic concept about treating all types of anxiety disorders
with cognitive therapy is to think of the patient as generally
making an effort to avoid something that is perceived as too

uncomfortable or dangerous. Patients who are anxious avoid specific situations, particular behavioral or physiological triggers, or even their own thoughts or emotional states (as in obsessive–compulsive disorder). Fear of shame and embarrassment can underlie the avoidance as in social phobia. The therapist must understand the patient's internal reality, including in what ways he or she avoids or engages in safety behaviors with his or her thinking, in order to conduct exposure-based treatment. Many patients with anxiety disorders have a propensity to use worry as a coping strategy in response to stress. Wells (2002) has furthered the conceptualization of cognitive therapy for anxiety disorders by building into the model the need for the therapist to aggressively target worry. The therapist helps the patient to look at his or her beliefs about the functional value of worry and the disadvantages of constant hypervigilance to decrease worry. Worry and rumination can be ways that patients avoid emotion and the possibility of being overwhelmed by a problem. Therapists can assign the patient to schedule his or her worry and thereby demonstrate that worry can be controlled.

MS. GREEN told the therapist "I'm a worrier" from the start and did not identify excess worry as a problem. She, in fact, thought of her worry as a positive trait—that worry made her a good mother, kept her from getting too upset about disappointing events, and helped her solve problems. Ms. Green's therapist began the process of educating Ms. Green about the relationship of her worry to her difficulties with anxiety. He slowly introduced experiments to refute the irrational ideas she had about worry. Ms. Green felt uncomfortable whenever she had strong emotional reactions to anything, and she would often use worry as a way to avoid her emotions. The therapist worked with Ms. Green to help her identify and manage her emotional states and increase her confidence and skill in her ability to solve problems. Ms. Green became upset and anxious whenever faced with a problem she needed to handle and generally worried and ruminated about the problem. She worked in therapy to identify the dysfunctional thoughts she had about problem solving ("If I make the wrong decision then it will be a disaster"). Her therapist taught her to identify a reasonable sequence of steps to be more effective in solving problems. The therapist assigned her weekly tasks to expose her to the process of actual problem solving, rather than to use worry and avoidance to manage difficulties.

Learning points

- Patients with anxiety disorders generally avoid situations, physiological triggers or thoughts, and emotional states. Exposure-based treatment interventions and cognitive restructuring are used in the cognitive therapy of anxiety disorders.
- Patients with panic disorder have catastrophic misinterpretation of physiological sensations leading to panic.
- Therapists treating anxiety disorders must attend to the safety behaviors patients use in order to truly conduct effective exposure; therapists must attend to worry and rumination.

REFERENCES

Barlow, D. H., Gorman, J. M., Shear, M. K., et al. (2000).Cognitive behavioral therapy, imipramine or their combination for panic disorder: A randomized controlled trial. *Journal of the American Medical Association. 283;* 2529–2536.

Barlow, D. H., & Cerny, J. A. (1988). *Psychological treatment of panic.* New York: The Guilford Press.

Beck, A. T., Emery, G., & Greenberg, R. (1985). *Anxiety disorders and phobias: A cognitive perspective.* New York: Basic.

Clark, D. M. (1986). A cognitive approach to panic. *Behavioral Research and Therapy. 24;* 461–470.

Clark, D. M. (1988) A cognitive model of panic. In S. Rachman & J. Maser (Eds.). *Panic: Psychological perspectives.* Hillsdale, NJ: Erlbaum.

Dobson, K. S. (Ed.). (2001). *Handbook of cognitive-behavioral therapies* (2nd ed.). New York: The Guilford Press.

Heimberg, R. G., & Becker, R. E. (2002). *Cognitive-behavioral group therapy for social phobia.* New York: The Guilford Press.

Salkovskis, P. M. (Ed.). (1996). *Frontiers of cognitive therapy.* New York: The Guilford Press.

Wells, A. (2002). *Emotional disorders and metacognition: Innovative cognitive therapy.* New York: John Wiley & Sons.

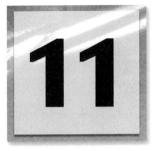

Personality Disorders and Dialectical Behavior Therapy

LEARNING OBJECTIVES

The reader will be able to:

1. Understand the basic model of personality disorders in cognitive therapy.
2. Modify the structure of cognitive therapy treatment to make it useful for personality disorders.
3. Know the basic features of dialectical behavior therapy (DBT) for borderline personality disorder.

Cognitive therapists modify the standard features of therapy when treating personality disorders. The basic principles of cognitive therapy—conceptualizing psychopathology as involving disturbances in thinking that lead to difficulties with mood and behavior, and that underlying beliefs lead to the primary disturbance in thinking—continue to be cornerstones of treatment. The conceptualization of personality disorders in cognitive therapy is that individuals with personality disorders develop dysfunctional interpersonal strategies to deal with other people and the world. These dysfunctional strategies may not differ from those used by individuals who do not have personality disorders, but they are dysfunctional because of their inflexible, inappropriate use and the inability of the patient to initiate more appropriate and functional behavior when it is clear that the strategies he or she is using are too costly. Individuals with personality disorders use particular behavioral strategies compulsively, even if they do not work in a given situation.

MS. GRAY consistently felt overwhelmed by her emotional responses, particularly when she felt ashamed or worthless. When she felt overwhelmed, her thoughts were generally that she "could not stand how she was feeling." When her therapist helped her to elaborate and explore this experience, he found that she meant that she thought she could not tolerate her feelings, developing escalating anxiety and a sense that she would "go crazy." When Ms. Gray was overwhelmed by her feelings, she would do anything to distract herself. She was generally in such a distraught state that the distraction techniques that she learned worked for her took extreme forms, like having physical fights, cutting herself, or overdosing. The consequence of the extreme behavior she used for distraction was the relief of her emotional tension (a reward). An additional consequence was that she frequently would get attention from other people and assistance with whatever problem precipitated her feeling worthless and ashamed. These consequences increased the probability of her using extreme behavior to manage her feelings in the future. Unfortunately, these extreme behaviors began to have significant serious consequences. Ms. Gray had several medical "close calls" and had "burned out" a number of her friends. Despite acknowledging these consequences, she felt she had "no control" over her behavior and had no other means of coping with her feelings.

Patients with personality disorders have painful core beliefs that are frequently activated and precipitate the use of compensatory strategies. Patients with personality disorders frequently have substantial skill deficits because the vicious cycle of overusing dysfunctional strategies keeps them from learning more adaptive behavior. The personality structures and interpersonal beliefs and strategies that cause difficulty are formed early in development and often are associated with early trauma or disruptions of attachment. Treatment often requires a substantial focus on developmental experiences and cognitive restructuring of those experiences.

One of **MS. GRAY's** core beliefs was "I'm bad and worthless." She also felt that it was intolerably painful to have this belief and that it was horribly shameful if other people knew how bad she was. To make certain other people didn't know she was worthless, she would pay selective attention to being ignored, because that would "prove" her

> worthlessness. When her boyfriend was preoccupied with preparing for an exam, she felt worthless and ashamed. Because she felt overwhelmed with shame, and unable to stand her feelings, she provoked him. They fought and she threw a glass at him. He called her crazy, and he stormed out of the house. This confirmed her belief about herself as worthless.

The core beliefs that personality-disordered patients develop are multidetermined. Childhood experiences can teach powerful negative messages, especially in extreme circumstances like abuse and neglect. Mismatches of child and parental styles and temperament or family belief systems can cause the patient to form a negative set of core beliefs. For example, a child who is bright and interested in education, and is born to parents of below-average achievement who disparage intellectual pursuits could develop negative beliefs about himself or herself and others.

> **MS. GRAY** was consistently belittled by her father. She also witnessed his verbal and physical abuse toward her mother. Her mother was frequently depressed and unavailable; she told Ms. Gray that it was impossible to cope with stress and that too much stress would make her go crazy. Her mother also said that she stayed with her father as long as she did because of Ms. Gray and her brother. Ms. Gray witnessed few examples of effective problem solving and effective interpersonal communication as a youngster. Besides feeling worthless because of her father's relentless barrage of criticism, Ms. Gray's mother dealt with stress by going to bed for days at a time, leaving Ms. Gray and her brother to fend for themselves. This lack of parental care and supervision added to Ms. Gray's sense of feeling overwhelmed. She would blame herself and feel worthless for not being able to cope more effectively or to help her mother more. She was ashamed of her family and would not bring friends home and constantly worried about people finding out how her family lived.

The therapist needs to develop a hypothesis about the development of the patient's core belief and share this with the patient. The therapist validates the patient's point of view by explaining that the core belief had an important purpose—that it was designed to make sense of childhood experiences and/or to protect the patient. The therapist makes a case for the core belief as now being less adaptive for the patient and that its rigidity would not allow the patient to develop alternative views with further life experience. The therapist slowly works to logically show the patient that the belief functions to process information and represents a problem for the patient. Gradually and empathically, he or she guides the patient to consider other possible beliefs, while remaining attuned to the patient's point of view. Frequently the therapist serves as a source of other possible perspectives to consider about the world or relationships, because the patient with a personality disorder has no other choice but to see the world in his or her own particular fashion.

 MS. GRAY began the work of understanding that she had a belief about herself being "bad" by refining her definitions of what "bad" meant and placing herself on a continuum of "bad." Her therapist had her construct a grid of good and bad people in the world and had her place herself on that grid. Despite this exercise, Ms. Gray remained prone to "feeling" that she was bad, and this feeling frequently instigated a cascade of emotions and behaviors that, at best, were difficult for her to bear, and at worst, precipitated self-harm. Since therapy initially involved teaching and motivating Ms. Gray to behave in less destructive ways, there were fewer instances of her behaving in a harmful fashion. Nevertheless, her "feelings were no different." Ms. Gray's therapist carefully explained to her how her belief that "I'm bad" worked like a screen, and that it filtered or distorted information so that she would continue to feel strongly that it was true—even if there was information to the contrary. The therapist also helped her to understand how prejudice is similar to this process, and that example made a real difference to Ms. Gray's understanding of why her feeling "bad" was so strong. Finally the therapist explained that a child in Ms. Gray's position would have little choice but to believe that the adults in her life were correct and that Ms. Gray had made sense of the chaos in her childhood by seeing herself as "bad and worthless." Ms. Gray was upset and looked sad at this moment.

The patient's thoughts and beliefs about the therapist play a significant role in the treatment of personality disorders. These ideas serve as data points that augment the conceptualization as well as to serve as opportunities to change core beliefs in session. Therapists need to be attuned to the alliance and to shifts in the patient's affect to take advantage of these opportunities.

The therapist noted the drop in **MS. GRAY'S** mood when he discussed Ms. Gray's core belief as originating from her attempt to make sense of her childhood experience. He asked her, "What's going through your mind?" She said, "I just feel so sad about it. I don't think I'll ever get over what happened." The therapist said that he agreed that painful circumstances happened to Ms. Gray in her daily life in childhood. He told her how sorry he was that she had dealt with such adversity. He asked her if she ever considered how people coped with terrible adversity. She was confused by his question. The therapist asked if she could think of examples of people who had survived calamities and what perspectives they developed to make sense of these. She could not think of anyone. The therapist asked if she knew about Christopher Reeve or Trisha Meili (the Central Park Jogger). They discussed together that each of these survivors had a choice after a devastating life event—to be a victim or to be a survivor. The therapist talked with Ms. Gray about how she, too, could make a choice to have a meaningful life despite having had a difficult and painful childhood. They began to look at what it would mean if she could think of herself in this way and how her life would be different. Ms. Gray was able to identify being in therapy, the progress she had made in not getting into fights, and getting her cutting behavior in better control as evidence of her "surviving." She identified her artwork as something that meant a great deal to her as a survivor. The therapist added that he knew that she had developed a relationship with her mother that was not like the relationship she had with her as a child. Ms. Gray acknowledged that her mother had changed "a lot" by being in therapy herself. Ms. Gray's therapist assigned her to record daily the evidence that she was working to build a meaningful and different life for herself.

Cognitive therapists often use role play and imagery in working with patients with personality disorders. Role play can identify skill deficits and help the patient to practice and develop new skills. Assertiveness and emotion regulation skills are often deficient in patients with personality disorders. Reverse role play, when the therapist plays the patient and the patient plays a significant person, can be a useful means of helping the patient to be more understanding about the experience of other people. After a trusting and well-grounded therapeutic relationship has been developed, role play can be used to reprocess and conceptualize early developmental experiences and to help the patient understand alternative explanations for the behavior of past significant figures. The therapist must make certain that there is sufficient time in the session and that the use of imagery and role play is well planned and explained; the therapist must be available to support the patient and process the experience at the end of the session. An excellent description of the use of this technique is contained in Judith Beck's book *Cognitive Therapy: Basics and Beyond*.

Imagery is another experiential technique useful for patients with personality disorders. Imagery can be used to restructure core beliefs about early developmental experiences and can be helpful in assisting patients to broaden the range of potential outcomes that exist regarding anxiety-provoking situations. Imagery can facilitate the discovery of fundamental core beliefs. The therapist helps the patient to remember pivotal developmental events in substantial detail. The therapist activates and inquires about core beliefs during critical negative developmental experiences. The therapist guides the patient through the image and suggests possible new ways to conceptualize or experience it. He or she works with the patient to form new beliefs by considering alternative explanations that were not available to him or her at the time of the negative experience. Patients can develop a wider frame of reference and empathy for others by conceptualizing the behavior of significant figures in the past—e.g., parents. Both role play and imagery have the added advantage of increasing the patient's affect, making substantive change more likely.

On several occasions, as **MS. GRAY** discussed her father's behavior when she was a child, Ms. Gray said, "I can just see him standing there, screaming at my mother." The therapist asked Ms. Gray if she was willing to work more with this image. She agreed. The therapist guided her through a detailed description of the situation and her thoughts and feelings as a child. The therapist frequently checked with Ms. Gray as to anxiety and mood in the present as they explored the image. When Ms. Gray got to the part in the image where she remembered feeling worthless, the therapist asked her, "As your adult self, what would you tell your child self about this situation?" Ms. Gray said, "Don't listen to him; you're just a little kid." She was visibly moved. This moment represented a turning point; it allowed her to consider alternative points of view about herself as well as to begin to understand her father's behavior.

Other particular techniques useful to therapists working with core beliefs in a patient with personality disorder, in addition to role play and imagery, include obtaining a detailed history and having the patient test the core belief for accuracy over a lifetime. Patients can identify facts about themselves that are not filtered by the core belief and change their self-evaluation. Using a cognitive continuum is another important technique in changing beliefs of patients with personality disorders. The patient learns to be less rigid and change dichotomous thinking when data is available that counters his or her perception of himself or herself or others (Chapter 5 gives examples of using these techniques).

Cognitive therapy with patients with personality disorders is longer in duration than cognitive therapy for many Axis I disorders. Treatment takes longer, in part, because of the need to pay particular attention to the development and maintenance of the therapeutic relationship. The therapeutic relationship needs to be strong and sufficiently trusting to allow the patient to identify dysfunctional strategies and beliefs and learn newer and more functional strategies. Since patients with personality disorders have, by definition, dysfunctional interpersonal strategies, the therapist must be creative, empathic, and patient. The process of forming a relationship is often gradual and fraught with difficulty. The therapist needs to teach the patient new ways of relating to other people and to help the patient to respond more rationally in relationships. The therapist can work first to help the patient deal with anxiety or depression, which engenders trust in the therapist and relationship, before tackling the harder task of dealing with dysfunctional beliefs and interpersonal strategies. Rapport and trust in the therapeutic relationship with these patients is often hard-won and slow to develop. Because patients have inflexible rules and dysfunctional interpersonal strategies, they often have a life filled with experiences to confirm their core beliefs, and only slowly form a therapeutic alliance.

MS. GRAY came 20 minutes late to her first three sessions. Her therapist directly addressed this, asking her what the problem was that kept her from coming on time. Ms. Gray was silent and looked visibly upset. The therapist asked Ms. Gray if she could talk about what thoughts and feelings she had about coming to therapy. Ms. Gray became quite angry and said, "I don't know how we will ever work together if you keep criticizing me." The therapist asked Ms. Gray if she could consider the advantages of coming to therapy on time and she said, "Great, now you think I'm stupid, too." The therapist told Ms. Gray that his primary concern was their relationship and solving the problem together.

> Ms. Gray and the therapist spent several minutes in each of the next two sessions working to solve the problem of Ms. Gray's lateness. He said there was no way he could control the time of Ms. Gray's arrival. They explored the advantages and disadvantages of coming on time, including that the therapist would be unable to be as helpful as if they had a full session. The therapist directly addressed that Ms. Gray could have no way of knowing if he could help her or if he would behave in a trustworthy manner. Eventually, Ms. Gray and the therapist brokered a compromise: she would make every effort to come on time, and the therapist would make every effort to be helpful. They would evaluate how therapy was progressing every session.

Therapy can stagnate if the therapist does not pay close attention to any variations in the patient's affect, to validating the patient's pain when dealing with difficult situations, or to confronting the patient's attempts to avoid pain. The therapist must acknowledge that therapy is a difficult and painful process that will ultimately help the patient to function better. The therapist must be direct in asking the patient for verbal feedback as well as exquisitely attuned to nonverbal feedback during the session. The therapist must make certain that the patient is capable of controlling self-destructive behavior before making efforts to use imagery and role play to change beliefs. Transference is used as a tool to understand the patient's beliefs. The therapeutic relationship often functions as a model for appropriate behavior in a real relationship. The therapist often must balance working on the goals of therapy and discussing more day-to-day issues. Active work to facilitate skill acquisition is critical.

Finally, the difficulty with engagement and treatment adherence for patients with personality disorders can stem from the thoughts and behaviors the therapist has toward the patient. The therapist must monitor his or her stance toward the patient and make certain it is empathic and nonjudgmental. This is easier to do if he or she does not think of the patient's dysfunctional interpersonal behavior as willful and personally directed. If the therapist can look at the value of dysfunctional behaviors to the patient, it is often easier to remain empathic. This concept—that dysfunctional behaviors make sense, given the patient's background and experience—when conveyed to the patient, often facilitates change. Because of destructive behavior and lack of trust, maintaining empathy is easier said than done in many situations.

Therapists who do not set adequate limits with patients will struggle with their own responses to patient behavior. Therapists can define the problem behaviors the patient has and problem solve with the patient how to avoid engaging in these behaviors, rather than have negative thoughts about the patient that damage therapy. Teaching the patient more skillful and effective behavior helps the therapeutic alliance and the patient's self-esteem. The therapist can identify and respond to patients' problem behaviors in a more effective way by obtaining supervision.

MS. GRAY made multiple suicide attempts by overdose. She cut herself repeatedly. Several therapists had thrown her out of treatment as a result of this behavior. One had told her she was "not able to be helped." She had heard emergency room personnel call her "manipulative" and "borderline." Ms. Gray's therapist wanted to make her self-harming behavior the first order of business. After an initial exploration of the value of looking at the problem and making a crisis card, the problem persisted, although in a less severe form. Ms. Gray would make veiled remarks about "having an out" and would often not return calls to the therapist after she phoned in a crisis.

The therapist was angry and anxious about Ms. Gray's behavior. In the next session, he put their relationship on the agenda to discuss. He told Ms. Gray that he had difficulty managing his anxiety about her safety and could not do his best work with her if she was unwilling to accept his help when she called for it. Furthermore, he told her that he was concerned that her commitment to stop harming herself was not strong enough. He asked if she had any ideas about how they could help her better handle the urge to harm herself. He said that he did not want to become a therapist who felt "burnt out" by her behavior and wanted her to live long enough to benefit from treatment. The therapist said he knew she behaved like this because she was in pain and that they needed to find less destructive ways for her to tolerate that pain. Ms. Gray agreed to make this a priority, and the therapist agreed to work consistently to help her manage her feelings.

DIALECTICAL BEHAVIOR THERAPY

In 1993, Marsha Linehan and colleagues at the University of Washington began to publish data about a modified cognitive behavioral therapy treatment for chronically suicidal patients with borderline personality disorder. The treatment was significantly effective at preventing suicidal behavior and decreasing the lethality of suicide and self-injurious behavior in these patients, as well as decreasing length and frequency of hospital stays and increasing treatment retention. There have been multiple subsequent studies replicating these findings, as well as studies about extending the use of the model to other disorders where impulse control is an issue (e.g., eating disorders). Dialectical behavior therapy (DBT) differs from standard cognitive therapy for personality disorders in the unique conceptualization it poses for the development of borderline personality, in the integration of acceptance and validation into the treatment, and in the staged approach it takes in the management of severely afflicted patients with both Axis I and Axis II disorders.

DBT advances a model for the development of borderline personality which states that the patient initially has a biological or temperamental predisposition to emotional dysregulation and then develops in a pervasively invalidating environment. In essence, patients with borderline personality begin as individuals who emotionally respond more rapidly to less intense stimuli with an inappropriate level of emotion, and with a harder time returning to baseline after they are emotionally triggered. This abnormal level of emotional response has the consequence of being extremely painful to the patient and interferes with learning and memory in interpersonal settings. The vulnerability to excess emotion is, by itself, insufficient for the development of the disorder. The other component that is necessary is that these emotionally vulnerable patients must then be raised in an environment that is pervasively invalidating of their private emotional experience. The invalidating environment can be as extreme as one which includes sexual, physical, or emotional abuse, or as subtle as the pervasive cultural message to "stop whining and snap out of it." In essence, patients are repeatedly shamed for their responses and not instructed in alternative and more functional ways of behaving and coping with emotional experience.

The result of the interaction between the invalidating environment and the vulnerability to excess emotion is that the patient is left in a state of chronic emotional dysregulation that feels intolerably painful. All of the criterion behaviors of borderline personality disorder are viewed as consequences of this emotional dysregulation—either as efforts that the patient makes to help regulate emotions or simply a manifestation of the emotional dysregulation itself. The basic paradigm is that the patient simply cannot tolerate how he or she is feeling and frantically seeks relief from that state.

The philosophical underpinnings of DBT that make it different from standard cognitive therapy techniques stem from Linehan's (1993) observation that using conventional cognitive behavioral techniques with chronically suicidal borderline patients was ineffective and led to noncompliance and treatment dropout. She observed that the mandate to change in therapy reproduced the invalidating environment experienced by these patients in their development. To balance this invalidation, she added acceptance and validation as a part of the therapeutic strategy. Acceptance in DBT is modeled after the form of radical acceptance as practiced by Eastern philosophical traditions. Validation is the active communication that the patient's perspective makes sense. Validation is a powerful tool that decreases shame and subsequently allows patients to consider alternative points of view. The therapist moves between the position of being an advocate and guide to help the patient to change, while simultaneously validating the patient's position by communicating an understanding of what wisdom exists in the patient's decisions and behavior. The important lesson of holding two perspectives at the same time counters dichotomous thinking. Self-acceptance and the need to change are seen as simultaneously valid. Validation does not mean endorsing damaging behaviors, but it means empathically communicating an understanding of the function of these behaviors in the context of the patient conceptualization. For example, the therapist might communicate to the patient an understanding that the purpose of overdosing might be to get some sleep and escape his or her feeling state and that the result of overdosing might be that people help him or her, so it would make sense that the patient would continue to overdose, even if it meant enduring the many negative consequences.

The patient is taught techniques of radical acceptance and mindfulness to increase emotional awareness and tolerance of feeling states while decreasing impulsive behavior. The model further uses dialectics as the philosophical construction, meaning that there is an emphasis on attempting to reach synthesis by moving between polarities and that change is accepted as a constant fact of life. This philosophy can be particularly helpful for a borderline patient who is attempting to resolve dichotomous thinking or to wrestle with unpleasant affects.

DBT is further distinguished by having specific hierarchies of treatment targets, with structured goals, stages, and treatment delivery modes. This structure is substantially important to decrease the chaos of treatment as usually delivered to these complex and challenging patients. Stage 1 of DBT, which is the part of treatment that has been most well studied, is designed with the goal of achieving a normal lifespan, obtaining a commitment to the therapeutic process, and reducing other behaviors that threaten the patient's health and safety. It lasts for 1 year, following a pretreatment phase designed to clearly obtain informed consent and commitment to therapy. The patient commits to the targets of treatment before therapy begins—namely, to work to stop suicidal and other self-injurious behaviors, to actively work on and maintain a commitment to therapy, and to reduce behaviors that interfere with his or her quality of life. During pretreatment the patient commits to an attendance policy of not missing either four consecutive therapy sessions or four consecutive skills groups. Should this attendance contract be broken, the patient is ineligible for therapy for 1 full year. The therapist and patient actively work to solve attendance problems—a frequent concern in working with borderline patients.

There are multiple modes of treatment delivery in DBT. The individual therapist typically meets with the patient once per week. The primary function of the individual therapist is to provide the patient with the motivation to behave differently and to help the patient to develop different contingencies to reinforce more functional and skillful behaviors. The therapist identifies cognitions, emotional states, and interpersonal consequences that keep the patient from behaving in a more functional way and helps the patient to develop alternatives to these obstacles. A basic tenet of DBT is that a powerful source of reinforcement for the patient is the relationship between the therapist and patient. The therapist uses this relationship to help the patient behave differently by reinforcing functional and adaptive behavior, modeling, coaching, and cheerleading when necessary. The therapist carefully monitors and manages the patient's emotional state in the session and helps the patient to use skills present or learned in skills training to avoid feeling overwhelmed. Patients are instructed to keep records of target behaviors (self-injurious behaviors/thoughts of self-harm, substance use, and so forth) as well as to record the skillful means by which they avoid engaging in these behaviors. The therapist and the patient proceed to work on specified treatment targets in a previously agreed-on order of priority—that is, suicidal/self-harming behaviors first, therapy-interfering behaviors second, and other quality-of-life-interfering behaviors third. Each instance of a target behavior is subjected to a behavioral analysis and a careful analysis of the antecedents and consequences of the behavior, as well as possible alternative ways to solve the problem without engaging in the behavior. The patient commits to try new, more functional behaviors in similar situations in the future. A variety of standard cognitive behavioral therapy methods including skills training, contingency management, cognitive modification and exposure, are flexibly employed to help the patient to engage in new behaviors.

DBT takes the change process one step further by adding another mode of service delivery. A main problem for patients with borderline personality disorder is that the patient often can acquire skills in therapy sessions but cannot generalize them to his or her natural environment. Therefore, an important mode of therapy delivery in DBT treatment is as needed phone coaching between the therapist and the patient. The phone calls are designed for the therapist to coach the patient in the use of new skills in difficult settings. The format is discussed with the patient in advance to teach the patient to use these phone contacts for coaching and skill acquisition. Phone calls can be scheduled or unscheduled, with one exception—that the therapist notifies the patient at the start of treatment that he or she will not engage in a telephone session with the patient if the patient has made any attempt at self-harm, except to ascertain that the patient has access to reasonable medical care. This feature of DBT corrects the iatrogenic reinforcement of borderline patients for self-injurious behavior—often the only time a therapist will accept an emergency call from a patient is when the patient has made an attempt to harm himself or herself. In DBT therapists respond to patients in crisis to provide reinforcement for them to employ different skills and more adaptively handle a crisis.

Two additional modes of service delivery exist in DBT. The first is skills training. Skills training is conducted in weekly, 2 ½-hour groups that the patient attends in addition to individual therapy. The mandate for patient attendance for skills training is similar to that of individual therapy—the patient cannot miss four consecutive sessions or he or she is dropped from all treatment and cannot return for a full year. The principle underlying the use of skills training groups is that patients who have borderline personality disorder are often extremely deficient in the psychological and self-management skills necessary to have a healthy life. This lack of skill development is conceptualized as a developmental delay—first, the emotional dysregulation that the patient experiences interferes with learning and memory necessary to acquire skills, and second, the patient frequently has grown up in an environment where skills were not modeled or were absent. Finally, many borderline patients subsequently have such traumatic lives that acquisition of new skills is impossible. The skills in DBT are taught in four rotating modules. They include acceptance-based skills (mindfulness, distress tolerance), and change-based skills (emotion regulation, interpersonal effectiveness). Patients are taught in skills training that distress is an unavoidable part of life and that by using more skillful means they will manage and tolerate it with fewer negative consequences. Skills that decrease vulnerability to excess emotion help the patient recognize and manage emotional states and increase their interpersonal effectiveness. The group is held specifically in a classroom setting to avoid the confusion between skill acquisition and group psychotherapy. Two group leaders are optimal. Specific efforts are made to make certain that patients have sufficient emotional control to acquire and practice the skill in class, avoid noncompliance with homework and group tasks, and leave the group each week in good emotional control.

The final mode of DBT service delivery is group consultation for the therapist. DBT is a team approach. It acknowledges that borderline patients present special challenges to therapists because the complexity of working with borderline patients can punish therapists for effective behavior and reinforce therapists for not behaving skillfully. Therapists need a team of supportive colleagues to support them in working with this difficult population of patients. Group consultation can decrease therapy-interfering behaviors by therapists.

The three stages of DBT that follow the successful completion of the acute phase of treatment (Stage 1) involve dealing with trauma (with a form of treatment that is akin in principle to Foa's [2001] cognitive behavioral treatment for posttraumatic stress disorder), managing problems in day-to-day work and relationships (with an approach similar to standard cognitive therapy), and finally, a phase of treatment that is designed to help the patient assimilate in an existential sense what has transpired in his or her life and develop the capacity for joy and freedom. Patients return to earlier phases of treatment based on clinical needs; it is not unusual, for example, in an early stage of recovery for a patient to redevelop suicidal thoughts and behaviors and to return to managing this according to the principles of Stage 1 DBT. The effectiveness of Stages 2 through 4 of DBT has yet to be tested, but rigorous study of Stage 1 has shown it to be a valuable tool to deal with a difficult group of patients.

Learning points

- Standard cognitive therapy methods are modified to treat patients with personality disorders, with greater alteration to the therapeutic alliance and to the developmental origin of core beliefs and dysfunctional interpersonal strategies.
- Childhood experiences often lead to the development of painful core beliefs and dysfunctional interpersonal strategies in personality disorders.
- Dialectical behavior therapy is a unique form of cognitive therapy designed to treat borderline personality disorder, with substantial data supporting its efficacy in treating self-harming behaviors and treatment attrition.

REFERENCES

Beck, A. T., Freeman, A., Davis, D. D., et al. (2003). *Cognitive therapy of personality disorders* (2nd ed.). New York: The Guilford Press.

Beck, J. S. (1995). *Cognitive therapy: Basics and beyond.* New York: The Guilford Press.

Foa, E.B., & Rothbaum, B.O. (2001). *Treating the trauma of rape: Cognitive behavioral therapy for PTSD.* New York: The Guilford Press.

Linehan, M. (1993). *Cognitive-behavioral treatment of borderline personality disorder.* New York: The Guilford Press.

Young, J., Klosko, J., & Weishaar, M. E. (2003). *Schema therapy: A practitioner's guide.* New York: The Guilford Press.

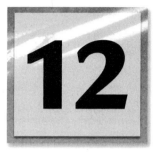

Medication Adherence

LEARNING OBJECTIVES
The reader will be able to:
1. Know data about combining psychopharmacological treatment with cognitive therapy.
2. Acquire tools from cognitive therapy that enhance medication adherence.
3. Understand particular beliefs that interfere with patients using medications properly.

Most therapists in clinical practice treat some patients who are managed with both medications and psychotherapy, and psychiatrists are likely to manage patients with medication who are in therapy with other providers. Cognitive therapy has proven to be an effective adjunct to treatment in two disorders traditionally treated primarily with medication—namely, schizophrenia (Kingdon & Turkington, 2005; Rector & Beck, 2001) and bipolar disorder (Lam, Jones, Hayward, & Bright, 1999). Cognitive therapy combined with medication increases the efficacy of treatment in severe and chronic major depression. Additionally, strategies taken from cognitive therapy improve adherence to medication treatment in several medical conditions—including diabetes and cardiovascular disease. Cognitive therapy has much to offer practitioners in assisting patients with medication adherence. Medication nonadherence is a substantial problem in psychiatric and medical disorders. Practitioners can provide patients with more effective means of dealing with chronic conditions by employing the tools of cognitive therapy. A valuable tool for challenging patients is cognitively conceptualizing the stumbling blocks to the effective use of medications.

An important caveat in combining cognitive therapy with medication is that truly combined treatment interventions have rarely been studied. Most studies involve medications provided in different settings and by different providers, rather than medications provided in an integrated way with therapy. Medications have the potential to have positive or negative effects on psychotherapy outcomes and vice versa. Existing studies indicate that in panic disorder and major depression, combined treatment with cognitive therapy and antidepressant medication is beneficial to treatment response (Wright, 2003). Studies of anxiety disorders combined with medication indicate that patients taking benzodiazepines do not respond to cognitive therapy treatment—effective exposure cannot occur with patients who are taking benzodiazepines, as they prevent anticipatory anxiety, forestall panic, and function as safety behaviors. Further studies of combined treatment may elucidate what sequence of treatment provides the most efficient and effective means of controlling symptoms and forestalling relapse.

Why do people not take medication as directed? Psychological issues and practical issues prevent all of us from taking medication as the prescriber intends. The practitioner who acknowledges his or her own difficulty with adhering to medication regimens will be far better equipped to understand and treat problems with medication adherence in his or her patients. Therapists who help patients to take medications more accurately will have far better outcomes because many patients who fail to take medication correctly have devastating results of nonadherence, particularly patients with affective disorders and schizophrenia.

Practical issues make it difficult for patients to take medication as the practitioner intends. This is the first area to remedy. The clinician must work to prescribe medication in the least complicated manner, including prescribing as few doses per day as is possible. Side effects must be regarded as a serious problem by the clinician and every step must be taken to try and restore the quality of life lost to the patient by his or her proper use of medication. The successful clinician will regard side effects as problems to be solved with the patient rather than dismiss them as something that the patient will just need to accept as a result of having an illness. Practical problems must always be solved in partnership with the patient. What does he or she think will help to increase the likelihood that medication will be remembered and taken? An astute clinician must remember that practical problems will vary from patient to patient—a 75-year-old patient with depression will likely have different issues from a 23-year-old college student with bipolar disorder.

The clinician who wants to maximize adherence to medications needs to help the patient to use behavioral reminders to help with adherence. Pill boxes with days of the week, notes on mirrors or refrigerators, associating taking medications with meals or bedtime, and using PDAs or electronic reminders are examples of strategies that increase the likelihood that patients will take medication as directed. Family members can be enlisted as partners to help patients with more severe disorders to remember to take medication, if the relationship allows for such assistance without undue exacerbation of conflict or increased expressed emotion in the family system. Patients should reward themselves for taking medications properly with positive self-statements or reinforcing activities.

Psychological obstacles that interfere with taking medications properly include alterations in the patient's mental state based on the illness itself, beliefs that the patient has, and forces from the patient's social network that can alter the motivation to comply with treatment (Beck, J., 2001).

Individuals with more severe psychiatric disorders have inherent obstacles to effectively taking medication. Patients with psychosis or severe mood disturbance have impairments in reality testing, problem solving, concentration, memory, and judgment. These impairments can themselves interfere with medication adherence. The therapeutic alliance with patients with severe mental disorders is critical. The clinician must evaluate the patient for specific mental status impairments that are barriers to adequate pharmacotherapy. The tools that cognitive therapy brings to the relationship with severely and persistently mentally ill patients are nonjudgmental and empathic assessment, relentless work to strengthen the therapeutic alliance, and a focus on problem solving and psychoeducation. The alliance is strengthened when the therapist actively assesses the patient's personal feelings about having the disorder and the use of medications. Advantage/disadvantage analyses about the pros and cons of using medication can help the patient to be a more effective partner. Therapists who explore the meaning of the illness to the patient and communicate respect for the patient's autonomy further the relationship and have better results. Clinicians who push to have patients take medications perfectly are less likely to be successful than clinicians who take a long view. If the therapist can determine what frequency of medication use is acceptable for the patient, and then examine the advantages and disadvantages of this frequency of medication use, then better adherence can occur.

Psychological problems with medication adherence often involve patient beliefs, and these beliefs are often amenable to cognitive therapy techniques. If confronting practical problems, educating the patient about his or her disorder and medications, processing the grief the patient has about having the disorder, and making certain that a positive therapeutic alliance exists proves ineffective, therapists should suspect beliefs as a factor in nonadherence. Beliefs that interfere with medication use come in several varieties, as described by Beck (2001). Patients have dysfunctional beliefs about physicians, about psychiatric illness, and about medications.

Cultural and interpersonal influences are significant mediators of beliefs that interfere with patients' medication adherence. Early learning about physicians, medications, and psychiatric illness has an enormous impact on the acceptance of psychotropic medication and psychiatric diagnoses. There is a pervasive cultural belief in the U.S. that strong and capable individuals solve problems without assistance or effort. The historical response to psychiatric illness in many cultures is to view it as a moral failing at best, and dangerous and demonic at worst. In the U.S., beliefs about physicians making patients "guinea pigs" and experimenting with medications on unsuspecting victims are culturally pervasive and have some basis in reality (e. g., Tuskegee). The media routinely portrays drug companies as foisting dangerous products on the public, and physicians as inept, avaricious, or criminal. Contrasting portrayals of "miracle cures," as well as the barrage of Internet information for which no quality control exists, influence patients' thinking about psychotropic drugs and prescribers.

Patients also have core beliefs about medications and physicians that are consistent with their cognitive style toward the world in general—a paranoid patient who believes that people in the world are likely to harm you is apt to regard his or her physician and prescribed medication with suspicion. Patients with personality disorders will frequently develop rigid beliefs and compensatory strategies toward medications and prescribing physicians similar to those that interfere with the other aspects of their lives.

Examining the patient's interfering beliefs, rules, and automatic thoughts for accuracy can improve medication adherence. The therapist can ask the patient to look at the evidence for a belief that "all people who take medication are weak." Patients must decrease the emotional reasoning they do about medications to be effective partners in treatment ("I know its not true that taking medication makes me weak, but I *feel* it is true"). Patients can do experiments with medication/lifestyle changes and evaluate outcomes to see if the predictions they make are accurate ("If I take my medication and don't drink and go to this party, I won't have any fun"). Finally, using principles of motivational interviewing and taking a future-oriented perspective can be of significant help to the patient ("If I want to finish college and get a job, how possible will that be if I continue to have manic episodes? What methods exist to prevent my manic episodes?"). Patients benefit from a clinician acknowledging that there is no "perfect" medication and no perfect adherence to medication treatment. Validating real difficulties with having mental illness without catastrophizing them, advocating for nondiscriminatory parity for psychiatric illness and problem solving, and normalizing grief about the significant losses facing patients all serve to enhance the therapeutic alliance and motivate patients to more diligently take medication.

The initial part of any cognitive therapy session with a patient on medications should include an adherence/medication side effect check as well as a mood or symptom check. Assessment of adherence early in the session demonstrates to the patient the critical nature of taking medication properly. How the clinician asks about adherence is as important as asking the question. Many clinicians will ask patients if they are taking medication regularly, and patients invariably answer, "Yes." Beginning clinicians will take the patient at his word or think the patient is lying, if it turns out to be untrue. A more realistic and comprehensive approach takes into account that patients are interested in appearing to be "good patients." The behavioral demand characteristics of the physician–patient relationship or therapist–patient relationship are such that patients often feel vulnerable and unequal and wish to please or not be seen as "bad" by the physician or therapist. This means patients will be unlikely to discuss problems with medication and adherence unless the clinician facilitates this discussion. First, the initial question to the patient needs to acknowledge that it is normal to have difficulty taking medication regularly (e. g., "How often have you been able to take your medication this week?" or "How much trouble have you had taking the medication this week?"). Second, the clinician needs to emphasize the benefits of medications as well as the side effects of medications in his or her inquiry. Frequently, patients are only asked about the bad effects medications have and are not reminded of the benefits of taking the medication. This has the unintended behavioral effect of reinforcing patients' belief that medication primarily has negative side effects and no benefits. Clinicians who balance questions like "Is the medication still helping you sleep better?" with "Have you noticed any weight gain from the medication?" are more likely to be successful, because they implicitly remind patients of the positive benefits of medication along with the less desirable effects.

Psychoeducation, a vital feature of cognitive therapy, is a core strategy to facilitate medication adherence. A critical element of this education involves assessing what the patient understands about the nature of his or her diagnosis and medications and correcting misconceptions. This education frequently dovetails with the need to help the patient to accept the diagnosis and to more accurately comprehend the meaning of the diagnosis and treatment. Severe psychiatric illnesses generally begin in young adulthood. The clinician must help the patient process grief about having a chronic life-changing disorder and assess the meaning of the disorder. The therapist must teach the patient about the illness, its symptoms, what medications can or cannot do, and what lifestyle changes he or she will need to make. When the patient has a diagnosis requiring long-term medication, clinicians must balance a discussion of the unwanted costs of the illness and the potential benefits of medication without necessarily touting taking medications as a desirable or positive event; acceptance of medication for many patients does not result in them feeling happy. Practitioners who had less desirable drug choices in terms of side effects in the past can fall prey to talking to patients about the "bad old days" when people "really suffered" with side effects, unlike at present; this attitude minimizes the real side effects of the current medication for the patient. Patients are often not "grateful" for scientific advances—what they would like is to not have the illness in the first place. Clinicians who help patients acknowledge their feelings of anger and grief about having the illness are more likely to have positive outcomes.

Cognitive therapy strategies can be used by clinicians who wish to improve care for patients who are constrained by insurance to briefer sessions. Even in a brief medication check, the therapeutic alliance is critical. Psychoeducation, activity scheduling, and thought records are all techniques that can be used by a clinician with limited time with a patient. The structure of cognitive therapy is efficient, prioritizes problems, and makes certain to obtain feedback, which benefits therapists in a setting where the 15-minute medication management check is the rule. Patients will feel more engaged and become better partners in their recovery.

Learning points

- Patients can have difficulties with practical and psychological problems that interfere with the use of medications.
- Cognitive therapy strategies can be beneficial for patients who are receiving medication treatment for psychiatric disorders.

REFERENCES

Basco, M. R., & Rush, A. J. (1996). *Cognitive-behavioral therapy for bipolar disorder*. New York: Guilford.

Beck, J. S. (2001). A cognitive therapy approach to medication compliance. In *Annual Review of Psychiatry*. Washington, D.C.: American Psychiatric Press.

Lam, D. H., Jones, S. H., Hayward, P., et al. (1999). *Cognitive therapy for bipolar disorder: A therapist's guide to concepts, methods and practice*. New York: John Wiley & Sons.

Kingdon, D., & Turkington, D. (2005). *Cognitive therapy of schizophrenia*. New York: Guilford Press.

Rector, N. A., & Beck, A. T. (2001). Cognitive behavioral therapy for schizophrenia: An empirical review. *Journal of Nervous Mental Diseases. 189;* 278–287.

Wright, J. H. (2003). Integrating cognitive therapy and pharmacotherapy. In Leahy, R. (Ed.) *New advances in cognitive therapy*. New York: The Guilford Press.

Wright, J. H., Thase, M. E., Beck, A. T., et al. (1993). *Cognitive therapy with inpatients: Developing a cognitive milieu*. New York: The Guilford Press.

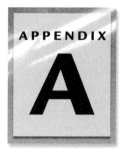

How Do I Become an Effective Cognitive Therapist?

"How do I become an effective cognitive therapist?" is a little like "How do I get to Carnegie Hall?" . . . Practice, practice, practice. Old jokes aside, one of the remarkable legacies of cognitive therapy is the data that exists about what works to train therapists in cognitive therapy and how to measure effective therapist adherence to the model. Three elements are necessary to train any therapist: didactic learning, patient care, and supervision. Therapists with inadequate amounts of any of these components think that they are more capable than they actually are in administering cognitive therapy (Kavanaugh, 1994). A common element in training relatively experienced therapists in cognitive therapy is that they require 20 to 30 hours of didactic training and 6 to 12 months of supervised clinical experience to become competent.

Fortunately, there are wonderful training opportunities in cognitive therapy. Residency training programs have started the process of adequately training residents. A number of cognitive therapy centers that provide training for professionals exist throughout the United States; a list of these centers is available on the Academy of Cognitive Therapy (ACT) web site: www. academyofct.org. Many forms of literature and educational media are available to the interested therapist. Therapists who engage in the process of consistently evaluating their effectiveness and seeking further training and supervision are likely to provide the best patient care; so competence is just the beginning.

The first part of learning to be a cognitive therapist involves establishing the relationship skills common to all good therapy and understanding the demands and boundaries of the therapeutic encounter. Therapists must read about and understand basic principles of human development and psychology. Therapists then learn the basic techniques of cognitive therapy: session structuring, the basic tools of treatment, models for specific disorders, and the beginning of conceptualization skills. Integrating conceptualization and treatment is a higher level skill, as is adapting the basic tenets of cognitive therapy to deal with more complicated problems.

A particular and important element of cognitive behavioral therapy is the tradition of measuring therapist competence. Young and Beck (1980) developed the Cognitive Therapy Scale (CTS) in order to determine if therapists were using the treatment competently. This scale determines both therapeutic integrity and the skillfulness with which the therapist employs the treatment with a particular patient. The scale has valid and reliable psychometric properties in trained raters. It has 11 items; each rated on a six-point scale. The scale measures both general therapeutic skills (i.e., understanding, collaborating, pacing) and specific cognitive therapy skills including guided discovery and the strategy chosen by the therapist to help the patient change. This scale is used in a number of ways. It provides researchers with a method that verifies the integrity of the treatment that they are testing; it can be used as a teaching tool or method to verify the competency of trainees; and it is used by the Academy of Cognitive Therapy as one part of the credentialing of certified cognitive therapy practitioners. It can be found, along with the manual detailing the scoring, on the Academy of Cognitive Therapy web site. The CTS is a valuable self-instruction tool as well as a wonderful teaching tool for trainees.

Finally, the Academy of Cognitive Therapy is an organization that can be extremely helpful to aspiring and established cognitive therapists. It was established in 1996 as a nonprofit organization with the purpose of assessing and certifying the competency of clinicians practicing cognitive therapy. Certification and membership offers clinicians the opportunity to further expand their knowledge through an active web-based list serve, used frequently by members to discuss educational, clinical, and research topics. ACT sponsors educational conferences and makes its members aware of other educational offerings in cognitive therapy both nationally and internationally.

REFERENCES

Dobson, K. S., Beck, J. S., & Beck, A. T. (2005). The Academy of Cognitive Therapy: Purpose, history and future prospects. *Cognitive and Behavioral Practice, 12,* 263–266.

Kavanaugh, D. J. (1994). Issues in multidisciplinary training of cognitive-behavioural interventions. *Behavior Change: Journal of The Australian Behavior Modification Association, 11*(3), 38–44.

Sudak, D. M., Beck, J. S., & Wright, J. S. (2003). Cognitive behavioral therapy: A blueprint for attaining and assessing psychiatric resident competency. *Academic Psychiatry, 27*(3), 154–159.

Vallis, T. M., Shaw, B. F., & Dobson, K. S. (1986). The cognitive therapy scale: Psychometric properties. *Journal of Consulting and Clinical Psychology, 54,* 31–38.

Young, J. E., & Beck, A. T. *The cognitive therapy scale.* Unpublished manuscript. Philadelphia: The University of Pennsylvania.

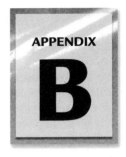

Case Formulation Guidelines and Example*

I. Case history (Suggested number of words: 750)
   General Instructions: The case history should briefly summarize the most important background information that is collected in evaluating the patient for treatment. Be succinct in describing the case history.
   A. Identifying information
      Provide a fictitious name to protect the confidentiality of patient. Use this fictitious name throughout the case history and formulation. Describe patient's age, gender, ethnicity, marital status, living situation, and occupation.
   B. Chief complaint
      Note chief complaint in patient's own words.
   C. History of present illness (HPI)
      Describe present illness, including emotional, cognitive, behavioral, and physiological symptoms. Note environmental stresses. Briefly review treatments (if any) that have been tried for the present illness.
   D. Past psychiatric history
      Briefly summarize past psychiatric history including substance abuse.
   E. Personal and social history
      Briefly summarize most salient features of personal and social history. Include observations on formative experiences, traumas (if any), support structure, interests, and use of substances.

* Reprinted with permission of the Academy of Cognitive Therapy.

F. Medical history

Note any medical problems (e.g., endocrine disturbances, heart disease, cancer, chronic medical illnesses, chronic pain) that may influence psychological functioning or the treatment process.

G. Mental status observations

List three to five of the most salient features of the mental status exam at the time treatment began. Include observations on general appearance and mood. Do *not* describe the entire mental status examination.

H. DSM IV diagnoses

Provide five Axis DSM IV diagnoses.

II. Case formulation (Suggested number of words: 500)

General Instructions: Describe the primary features of your case formulation using the following outline.

A. Precipitants

Precipitants are large-scale events that may play a significant role in precipitating an episode of illness. A typical example is a depressive episode precipitated by multiple events, including failure to be promoted at work, death of a close friend, and marital strain. In some cases (e.g., bipolar disorder, recurrent depression with strong biological features) there may be no clear psychosocial precipitant. If no psychosocial precipitants can be identified, note any other features of the patient's history that may help explain the onset of illness.

The term *activating situations*, used in the next part of the case formulation, refers to smaller-scale events and situations that stimulate negative moods or maladaptive bursts of cognitions and behaviors. For example, the patient who is depressed following the precipitating events described above may experience worsening of his or her depressed mood when he or she is at work, or when he or she is with spouse, or when he or she attends a class he or she used to attend with a friend who died.

Which *precipitants* do you hypothesize played a significant role in the development of the patient's symptoms and problems?

B. Cross-sectional view of current cognitions and behaviors

The *cross-sectional* view of the case formulation includes observations of the predominant cognitions, emotions, and behaviors (and physiological reactions if relevant) that the patient demonstrates in the "here and now" (or demonstrated prior to making substantive gains in therapy). Typically the cross-sectional view focuses more on the surface cognitions (i.e., automatic thoughts) that are identified earlier in therapy than underlying schemas, core beliefs, or assumptions that are the centerpiece of the *longitudinal* view described below.

The *cross-sectional* view should give a conceptualization of how the cognitive model applied to this patient early in treatment. List up to three current activating situations or memories of activating situations. Describe the patient's typical automatic thoughts, emotions, and behaviors (and physiological reactions if relevant) in these situations.

C. Longitudinal view of cognitions and behaviors
This portion of the case conceptualization focuses on a *longitudinal* perspective of the patient's cognitive and behavioral functioning. The *longitudinal view* is developed fully as therapy proceeds, and the therapist uncovers underlying schemas (core beliefs, rules, assumptions) and enduring patterns of behavior (compensatory strategies).

What are the patient's key schemas (core beliefs, rules, or assumptions) and compensatory behavioral strategies? For patients whose premorbid history was not significant (e.g., a bipolar patient with no history of developmental issues that played a role in generation of maladaptive assumptions or schemas), indicate the major belief(s) and dysfunctional behavioral patterns present only during the current episode. Report developmental antecedents relevant to the origin or maintenance of the patient's schemas and behavioral strategies or offer support for the hypothesis that the patient's developmental history is not relevant to the current disorder.

D. Strengths and assets
Describe in a few words the patient's strengths and assets (e.g., physical health, intelligence, social skills, support network, work history, etc.).

E. Working hypothesis (summary of conceptualization)
Briefly summarize the principal features of the working hypothesis that directed treatment interventions. Link the working hypothesis with the cognitive model for the patient's disorder(s).

III. Treatment plan (Suggested number of words: 250)
General Instructions: Describe the primary features of the treatment plan using the following outline.
   A. Problem list
      List any significant problems that you and the patient have identified. Usually problems are identified in several domains (e.g., psychological/psychiatric symptoms, interpersonal, occupational, medical, financial, housing, legal, and leisure). Problem lists generally have two to six items, sometimes as many as eight or nine items. Briefly describe problems in a few words, or, if previously described in detail in the HPI, just name the problem here.
   B. Treatment goals
      Indicate the goals for treatment that have been developed collaboratively with the patient.
   C. Plan for treatment
      Weaving together these goals, the case history, and the working hypothesis, briefly state your treatment plan for this patient.
IV. Course of treatment (Suggested number of words: 500)
General Instructions: Describe the primary features of the course of treatment using the following outline.
   A. Therapeutic relationship
      Detail the nature and quality of the therapeutic relationship, any problems you encountered, how you conceptualized these problems, and how you resolved them.
   B. Interventions/procedures
      Describe three major cognitive therapy interventions you used, providing a rationale that links these interventions with the patient's treatment goals and your working hypothesis.
   C. Obstacles
      Present one example of how you resolved an obstacle to therapy. Describe your conceptualization of why the obstacle arose, and note what you did about it. If you did not encounter any significant obstacles in this therapy, describe one example of how you were able to capitalize on the patient's strengths in the treatment process.
   D. Outcome
      Briefly report on the outcome of therapy. If the treatment has not been completed, describe progress to date.

CASE WRITEUP EXAMPLE[†]

December 2, 1998
  I. Case history [Actual word count: 774] (Suggested number of
     words: 750)
     A. Identifying information
        Ann is a 44-year-old, twice-divorced, Caucasian woman
        who has no children, lives alone, and has been working
        full-time as a Spanish teacher for the past 22 years.
     B. Chief complaint
        Ann sought treatment due to an escalation in her depres-
        sion which started in October, 1996. She reported that she
        was also binge eating and overusing and abusing laxatives
        at least once a week, though she was much more con-
        cerned by the depression than the eating/laxative problem.
     C. History of present illness
        In October, 1996, Ann divorced her second husband and
        began to develop depressive symptoms (sadness, crying,
        social withdrawal, severe self-criticism). The depression
        worsened until it reached the severe level in March,
        1997. At intake (May, 1997), her symptoms included the
        following: emotional symptoms: sadness, anxiety, lack of
        interest in almost all activities; cognitive symptoms: diffi-
        culty concentrating, believing she was worthless and
        unlovable; behavioral symptoms: crying, social isolation;
        and physiological symptoms: difficulty falling asleep,
        tiredness.
            She developed sub clinical symptoms of bulimia ner-
        vosa in April, 1997. At intake, she reported that she
        binged, felt out of control of this behavior, and overused
        laxatives about once a week; she was (and is) intermit-
        tently preoccupied with a misperception that she is fat and
        is highly self-critical.
            The major stressors in Ann's life are social ones. Since
        her divorce she has withdrawn from friends, family, and
        co-workers. She has dated several times since her di-
        vorce, but each date has been a one-night stand, which
        leaves her feeling rejected and defective. She used to

---

[†] Reprinted with permission of the Academy of Cognitive Therapy.

derive significant satisfaction from relationships but has isolated herself and now feels sad, lonely, and rejected by others. While she finds it more difficult to do her job, work does not appear to be a significant stressor.

Ann restarted Prozac about 2 weeks ago (prescribed by her family physician) but thus far sees no change in her depressive symptoms.

D. Psychiatric history

Ann's first episode of major depression occurred in 1977 when her first husband divorced her. She was hospitalized for three weeks and was given Elavil. She discontinued the medication (against medical advice) at discharge but initiated psychological treatment (cognitive therapy) for the first time. Her depression remitted after 4 months of this outpatient psychotherapy, though she remained in therapy on a biweekly basis for another year, working on Axis II issues.

In 1989, Ann and her second husband received about six sessions of (predominantly psychodynamic) marital counseling which she found "mildly helpful."

In October, 1996, Ann's family physician prescribed Prozac, which initially helped reduce her depressive symptoms. The depression worsened in December, 1997, and she discontinued the medication on her own.

E. Personal and social history

Ann grew up the middle child of three. Her parents were Italian immigrants and her mother did not speak English. Ann considered herself the "ugly duckling" of the family. Her older sister was considered thin and pretty while Ann was called "chubette" and "big nose." She felt as if she were an extra burden to her family since they strongly wanted a boy when she was born. Her younger brother was born 18 months later and received nearly all the family's attention. She describes her father as having been strict, controlling, demanding, and concerned about what others thought of him. She describes her mother as quiet, unhappy, not affectionate, and old-fashioned. Ann felt unloved and unable to measure up to her siblings.

Ann attended Catholic school where she reports being trained to be "the perfect soldier." She married for the first time at age 18. She reports that she was abused and controlled by her first husband, who was violent at times. She believed she deserved the abuse and submitted to his wrath. When she finally got the courage to leave the marriage, she did not have her family's approval and to this day resents their lack of support.

Ann remarried in 1989. Her second husband reportedly spent a lot of time with young men, and Ann suspects he was bisexual. He ceased having any sexual relations with her about 3 years after their marriage. Though they tried marriage counseling briefly, her husband was unwilling to work on modifying the situation and they divorced in October of 1996.

F. Medical history

Ann did not have any medical problems which influenced her psychological functioning or the treatment process.

G. Mental status check

Patient is fully oriented with depressed mood.

H. DSM IV diagnoses

Axis I: Major depressive episode, recurrent, severe; Rule out bulimia nervosa

Axis II: Avoidant personality disorder

Axis III: None

Axis IV: Divorce; multiple relationship failures

Axis V: GAF current—68. Best in past year—80.

II. Case formulation [Actual word count: 403] (Suggested number of words: 500)

A. Precipitants

Ann's second divorce probably precipitated a recurrence of depression. Although it was she who initiated the divorce, she nevertheless felt rejected, believing that if she were more lovable, her husband would have fought to save the relationship. Feeling not only unloved by and unlovable to her husband but also unlovable in general, she began to isolate herself. She was no longer getting much positive input from her friends, family, and co-workers because of her lack of contact with them. But, like the divorce, she perceived this self-initiated reduction of contact as their rejecting her, instead of her withdrawing from them. She became increasingly sad and lonely and other depressive symptoms began to develop.

B. Cross-sectional view of current cognitions and behaviors
A typical current problematic situation is that Ann has just had sex on the first date with a man. Lying in bed with him she has the automatic thoughts, "I'm so ugly. What does he see in me? He'll never call; I might as well get up and leave now." Emotionally she feels sad and her behavior is to leave abruptly (probably appearing unfriendly, at best, to her date). A second typical situation is that she's reflecting on how a man has not called her back after a date. Her automatic thoughts are, "I'm too fat. No one wants me." She then feels sad, binges, and takes laxatives. A third situation is attending a family dinner where she perceives her father as being critical about her and her mother as lacking affection. She thinks, "No one cares about me; there's something wrong with me. I'm unimportant." She feels sad and becomes monosyllabic, speaking only when spoken to.

C. Longitudinal view of cognitions and behaviors
Ann grew up with non-English speaking Italian immigrant parents: a father who was demanding and critical and a mother who was emotionally distant. Early on she developed the belief that she was defective and unlovable. These beliefs were strengthened by the attention heaped on her younger brother, by increasing academic expectations of her father, by the criticisms of her teachers, and by her self-comparisons to her more attractive older sister. She developed the following key assumption: "If I'm perfect, don't cause trouble, and try always to please others, they'll like me. If I don't, they'll find me unlovable." Her compensatory behavioral strategies included being overly compliant, submissive, "perfectly" behaved, and avoidant of conflict.

D. Strengths and assets
Ann has had many years of success in her professional life. In her role as teacher, she is extremely well liked by her students, and given high praise from her peers.

E. Working hypothesis (summary of conceptualization)
It is understandable that Ann came to view herself as unlovable and defective as a result of the circumstances of her childhood. Being the daughter of highly demanding, critical European parents, her strict parochial education,

and her abusive marriages, laid the foundation and then reinforced her negative view of herself. This negative self-view is typically activated in interpersonal situations where she perceives rejection.

In order to function in the world, she has established rigid assumptions for herself: i.e., "I must be perfect or people will reject me," "I must please others, or they will dislike me." To operationalize her assumptions, she has developed the following behavioral compensatory strategies: submission, avoidance, and acquiescence.

III. Treatment plan [Actual word count: 195] (Suggested number of words: 250)

A. Problem list
  1. "Ann bashing"—hating self (ugly and unlovable).
  2. Depression; especially loneliness, sadness, crying.
  3. Avoidance and isolation: wanting to be loved but fearing rejection.
  4. Anxiety: fearing serious consequence of unrelenting depression.
  5. Binge eating and abuse of laxatives.
  6. Resentment toward parents for lack of affection and love.

B. Treatment goals
  1. Reduce dysfunctional behaviors: verbally berating herself; bingeing and purging; and isolation.
  2. Reduce negative distorted thinking.
  3. Increase self-worth, self-value, and self-image. (Modify unlovability and not-good-enough [defective] schemas).
  4. Find healthier ways to have fun.
  5. Gain confidence to go out alone and take risks in pursuing intimacy again.
  6. Build assertiveness skills and reduce subjugation.

C. Plan for treatment
The treatment plan was to reduce Ann's depression through helping her respond to her automatic thoughts (especially those connected with unlovability) and activity scheduling (especially to increase socializing). We also worked on alternative behaviors to bingeing when she was upset. Next, we tested her assumptions about being rejected if she displeased people and then worked on

assertiveness skills. We are currently working at the belief level, modifying her view of herself as unlovable and defective.

IV. Course of treatment [Actual word count: 300] (Suggested number of words: 500)

A. Therapeutic relationship

Treatment was facilitated by Ann's eagerness to please ("If I please others, they'll like me") but the counterpoint to this assumption ("If I disagree with people, they won't [like me]") did interfere slightly. Ann was too eager to please in therapy; she quickly agreed with me, sometimes without really stopping to reflect on the hypotheses or alternative perspectives I presented to her. I was able to elicit from her another belief ("If I tell someone I disagree, they'll take it as criticism"), helped her test these beliefs with me, correct her thinking, and then she became more willing to tell me when she didn't fully understand or agree with what I had said.

B. Interventions/procedures

1. Taught patient standard cognitive tools of examining and responding to her automatic thoughts (which allowed the patient to see her dysfunctional distorted logic and thus significantly reduced depressive and anxious symptoms).

2. Had Ann conduct behavioral experiments to test her assumptions (e.g., "If I say no to a man about having sex on a first date, he'll get mad and never call me again."). This resulted in reduced avoidance and increased assertiveness.

3. Had Ann keep an ongoing log of evidence that she was a loveable person, which helped her modify a key core belief.

B. Obstacles

When Ann had a bad week, she became hopeless about therapy. We reframed her setback as a reactivation of her schema due to an unfortunate incident with a date and as an opportunity to practice responding to negative automatic thoughts and solidifying a new, healthier belief.

D. Outcome

After starting therapy, Ann's depression gradually reduced over a 4-month period, until she was in full remission. She remains in therapy to work on lingering problems with male relationships and her self-image.

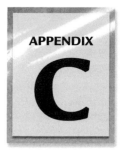

Academy of Cognitive Therapy Reading List*

THERAPY AND RESEARCH

Alford, B. A., & Beck, A. T. (1997). *The integrative power of cognitive therapy.* New York: Guilford Press.

Asmundson, G. J. G., Taylor, S., & Cox, B. J. (Eds.). (2001). *Health anxiety: Clinical and research perspectives on hypochondriasis and related disorders.* Chichester, England: John Wiley & Sons, Inc.

Beck, A. T. (1999). *Prisoners of hate: The cognitive basis of anger, hostility, and violence.* New York: Harper Collins Publishers.

Beck, A. T. (1999). Cognitive aspects of personality disorders and their relation to syndromal disorders: A psychoevolutionary aspect. In Cloninger, C. R. (Ed.), *Personality and psychopathology.* Washington, D.C.: American Psychiatric Press.

Butler, A. C., & Beck, J. S. (2000). Cognitive therapy outcomes: A review of meta-analyses. *Journal of the Norwegian Psychological Association, 37,* 1–9.

Clark, D. A., Beck, A. T., & Alford, B. A. (1999). *Scientific foundations of cognitive therapy and therapy of depression.* New York: John Wiley & Sons, Inc.

Gelder, M. (1997). The scientific foundations of cognitive behavior therapy. In Clark, D. M., & Fairburn, C. G. (Eds.), *Science and practice of cognitive behaviour therapy* (pp 27–46). New York: Oxford University Press, Inc.

Hollon, S. D., & Beck, A. T. (1994). Cognitive and cognitive-behavioral therapies. In M. J. Lambert (Ed.), Bergin and Garfield's *Handbook of Psychotherapy and Behavior Change* (5th ed., pp. 447–492). New York: John Wiley & Sons, Inc.

*A complete list, including non-English readings, is available at www.academyofct.org.
Reprinted with permission of Judith S. Beck.

Holmes, E. A., & Hackmann, A. (Eds.). (2004). *Mental imagery and memory in psychopathology.* London: Psychology Press, Taylor and Francis Group.

Ingram, R. E., Miranda, J., & Segal, Z. V. (1999). *Cognitive vulnerability to depression.* New York: Guilford Press.

Leahy, R. L. (Ed.). (2004). *Contemporary cognitive therapy: Theory, research, and practice.* New York: Guilford Press.

Leahy, R. L. (2003). *Psychology and the economic mind: Cognitive processes and conceptualization.* New York: Springer Publishing Company.

Neenan, M., Dryden, W., & Dryden, C. (2000). *Essential cognitive therapy.* Whurr Publications Limited.

Papageorgiou, C., & Wells, A. (2003). *Depressive rumination: Nature, theory and treatment.* New York: John Wiley & Sons.

Rosner, J. (2002). *Cognitive therapy and dreams.* New York: Springer Publishing Company.

Taylor, S. (Ed.). (1999). *Anxiety sensitivity: Theory, research, and treatment of the fear of anxiety.* Mahwah, NJ: Lawrence Erlbaum Associates.

Taylor, S. (Ed.). (2004). *Advances in the treatment of posttraumatic stress disorder: Cognitive-behavioral perspectives.* New York: Springer Publishing Company.

Wright, J. (Ed.). (2004). *Cognitive-behavior therapy.* (REVIEW OF PSYCHIATRY). Washington, D.C.: American Psychiatric Press.

CLINICAL APPLICATIONS: GENERAL

Beck, J. S. (1995). *Cognitive therapy: Basics and beyond.* New York: Guilford Press.

Dobson, K. S. (Ed.). (1999). *Handbook of cognitive-behavioral therapies* (2nd ed.). New York: Guilford Press.

Freeman, A., Pretzer, J., Fleming, B. (Ed.). (2004). *Clinical applications of cognitive theory* (2nd. ed.). New York: Plenum Publishers.

Freeman, S. M., & Freeman, A. (Eds.). (2005). *Cognitive behavior therapy in nursing practice.* New York: Springer Publishing Company.

Ledley, D. R., Marx, P., & Heimberg, R. G. (2005). *Making cognitive-behavioral therapy work: clinical process for new practitioners.* New York: Guilford Press.

Leahy, R. L. (2003). *Cognitive therapy techniques: A practitioner's guide.* New York: Guilford Press.

Ludgate, J. W. (1995). *Maximizing psychotherapeutic gains and preventing relapse.* Sarasota, FL: Professional Resource Press.

McMullin, R. E. (1999). *The new handbook of cognitive therapy techniques.* New York: W.W. Norton Co.

Needleman, L. D. (1999). *Cognitive case conceptualization: A guidebook for practitioners.* Mahwah, NJ: Lawrence Erlbaum Associates.

Nezu, A., Nezu, C. M., & Lombardo, E. (2004). *Cognitive-behavioral case formulation and treatment design: A problem-solving approach.* New York: Springer Publishing Co.

O'Donohue, W., Fisher, J., & Hayes, S. (2004). *Cognitive behavior therapy: Applying empirically supported techniques in your practice.* New York: John Wiley & Sons, Inc.

Padesky, C. A., & Greenberger, D. (1995). *Clinician's guide to mind over mood.* New York: Guilford Press.

Persons, J. B. (1989). *Cognitive therapy in practice: A case formulation approach.* New York: Norton.

Schuyler, D. (2003). *Cognitive therapy: A practical guide.* W. W. Norton & Company.

Wells, A. (2002). *Emotional disorders and metacognition: Innovative cognitive therapy.* New York: John Wiley & Sons, Inc.

CLINICAL APPLICATIONS: BOOKS ON SPECIFIC DISORDERS, PROBLEMS, OR POPULATIONS

ANXIETY DISORDERS

Antony, M. M., & Swinson, R. P. (2000). *Phobic disorders and panic in adults: A guide to assessment and treatment.* Washington, D.C.: American Psychological Association.

Beck, A. T., Emery, G., & Greenberg, R. (1985). *Anxiety disorders and phobias: A cognitive perspective.* New York: Basic.

Clark, David A. (2004). *Cognitive-behavioral therapy for OCD.* New York: Guilford Press.

Foa, E. B., & Rothbaum, B. O. (2001). *Treating the trauma of rape: Cognitive-behavioral therapy for PTSD.* New York: Guilford. (Original work published 1997.)

Follette, V. M., Ruzek, J. I., & Abueg, F. R. (1998). *Cognitive-behavioral therapies for trauma.* New York: Guilford Press.

Frost, R. O., & Steketee, G. (Eds.). (2002). *Cognitive approaches to obsessions and compulsions: Theory, assessment, and treatment.* Elmont, NY: Pergamon Press.

Heimberg, R. G., & Becker, R. E. (2002). *Cognitive-behavioral group therapy for social phobia.* New York: Guilford Press.

Najavits, L. M. (2001). *Seeking safety: A treatment manual for PTSD and substance abuse.* New York: Guilford Press.

Rygh, J. R., & Sanderson, W. C. (2004). *Treating generalized anxiety disorder: Evidence-based strategies, tools, and techniques.* New York: Guilford Press.

Taylor, S. (2000). *Understanding and treating panic disorder: Cognitive-behavioural approaches.* New York: John Wiley & Sons, Inc.

Taylor, S., & Asmundson, G. J. G. (2004). *Treating health anxiety: A cognitive-behavioral approach.* New York: Guilford.

Taylor, S. (2004). *Advances in the treatment of posttraumatic stress disorder: Cognitive-behavioral perspectives.* New York: Springer Publishing Company.

Woods, D., & Miltenberger, R. (Eds.). (2001). *Tic disorders, trichotillomania, and other repetitive behavioral disorders: Behavioral approaches to analysis and treatment.* Kluwer Academic Press.

BIPOLAR DISORDER

Basco, M. R., & Rush, A. J. (1996). *Cognitive-behavioral therapy for bipolar disorder.* New York: Guilford Press.

Johnson, S. L., & Leahy, R. L. (Eds.). (2003). *Psychological treatment of bipolar disorder.* New York: Guilford Press.

Lam, D. H., Jones, S. H., Hayward, P., & Bright, J. A. (1999). *Cognitive therapy for bipolar disorder: A therapist's guide to concepts, methods and practice.* New York: John Wiley & Sons, Inc.

Newman, C. F., Leahy, R. L., Beck, A. T., Reilly-Harrington, N. A., & Gyulai, L. (2002). *Bipolar disorder: A cognitive therapy approach.* Washington, D.C.: American Psychological Association.

CHILDREN

Albano, A. M., & Kearney, C. A. (2000). *When children refuse school: A cognitive behavioral therapy approach: Therapist guide.* Psychological Corporation.

Allen, J. S., & Christner, R. W. (2003, Fall). The process and structure of cognitive-behavior therapy (CBT) in the school setting. *Insight, 24* (1), 4–9.

Braswell, L., & Bloomquist, M. L. (1991). *Cognitive-behavioral therapy with ADHD children: Child, family, and school interventions.* New York: Guilford Press.

Christner, R. W., & Allen, J. S. (2003, Spring). Introduction to cognitive-behavioral therapy (CBT) in the schools. *Insight, 23* (3), 12–14.

Deblinger, E. & Heflin, A. H. (1996). *Treating sexually abused children and their nonoffending parents: A cognitive behavioral approach.* Thousand Oaks, CA: Sage Publications.

Dudley, C. D. (1997). *Treating depressed children: A therapeutic manual of cognitive behavioral interventions.* Oakland, CA: New Harbinger Publications.

Edelman, S., & Remond, L. (2004). *Taking charge! A guide for teenagers: Practical ways to overcome stress, hassles and upsetting emotions*. St. Leonards, Australia: Foundation for Life Sciences.

Epstein, N. E., Schlesinger, S. E., & Dryden, W. (Eds.). (1988). *Cognitive-behavioral therapy with families*. New York: Brunner-Mazel.

Friedberg, R. D., & Crosby, L. E. (2001). *Therapeutic exercises for children: Professional guide*. Sarasota, FL: Professional Resource Press.

Friedberg, R. D., Friedberg, B. A., & Friedberg, R. J. (2001). *Therapeutic exercises for children: Guided self-discovery using cognitive-behavioral techniques*. Professional Resource Exchange.

Friedberg, R., & McClure, J. (2001). *Clinical practice of cognitive therapy with children and adolescents: The nuts and bolts*. New York: Guilford Press.

Graham, P. (1998). *Cognitive-behaviour therapy for children and families*. Cambridge, England: Cambridge University Press.

Kazdin, A. E., & Weisz, J. R. (Eds.). (2003). *Evidence-based psychotherapies for children and adolescents*. New York: Guilford Press.

Keat, D. (1990). *Child multimodal therapy*. NJ: Ablex Publishing Corporation.

Kendall, P. C. (Ed.). (2000). *Child and adolescent therapy: Cognitive-behavioral procedures* (2nd ed.). New York: Guilford Press.

Kendall, P. C., Chansky, T. E., Kane, M. T., Kim, R. S., Kortlander, E., Ronan, K. R., et al. (1992). *Anxiety disorders in youth: Cognitive behavioral interventions*. Boston, MA: Allyn & Bacon.

Knell, S. M. (1993). *Cognitive behavioral play therapy*. Northvale, NJ: Jason Aronson, Inc.

March, J. S., & Mulle, K. (1998). *OCD in children and adolescents: A cognitive-behavioral treatment manual*. New York: Guilford Press.

Mennuti, R., & Christner, R. W. (in press). A conceptual framework for school-based cognitive-behavior therapy. In A. Freeman (Ed.), *International Encyclopedia of Cognitive Behavior Therapy*. New York: Kluwer.

Rapee, R., Wignall, A., Hudson, J., & Schniering, C. (2000). *Treating anxious children and adolescents: An evidence-based approach*. Oakland, CA: New Harbinger Publications.

Reinecke, M. A., Dattilio, F. M., & Freeman, A., (Eds.). (2003). *Cognitive therapy with children and adolescents: A casebook for clinical practice*. (2nd ed.). New York: Guilford Press.

Riley, D. (1997). *The defiant child: A parent's guide to oppositional defiant disorder*. Dallas: Taylor Publishing Company.

Ronen, T. (1997). *Cognitive developmental therapy with children*. New York: John Wiley & Sons, Inc.

Schwebel, A., & Fine, M. (1994). *Understanding and helping Families: A cognitive-behavioral approach*. Mahwah, NJ: Lawrence Erlbaum Associates.

Seligman, M. P., Reivich, K., Jaycox, L., & Gillham, J. (1995). *The optimistic child*. Boston, MA: Houghton Mifflin Co.

Stallard, P. (2002). *Think good—feel good: A cognitive behaviour therapy workbook for children.* Halsted Press.

Tanguay, P. (2001). *Nonverbal learning disabilities at home: A parent's guide.* Philadelphia: Jessica Kingsley Publishers.

Temple, S. D. (1997). *Brief therapy of adolescent depression.* Sarasota, FL: Professional Resources Press.

U.S. Department of Education. (2001). *Twenty-third annual report to Congress on the implementation of the Individuals with Disabilities Education Act.* Washington, D.C.

U.S. Department of Health and Human Services. (1999). *Mental health: A report of the Surgeon General.* Rockville, MD.

Wilkes, T. C. R., Belsher, G., Rush, A. J., & Frank, E. (1994). *Cognitive therapy for depressed adolescents.* New York: Guilford Press.

DEPRESSION AND SUICIDE

Beck, A. T., Rush, A. J., Shaw, B. F., & Emery, G. (1979). *Cognitive therapy of depression.* New York: Guilford Press.

Freeman, A., & Reinecke, M. (1994). *Cognitive therapy of suicidal behavior.* New York: Springer Publishing Company.

McCullough, J. P. (1999). *Treatment for chronic depression: Cognitive behavioral analysis system of psychotherapy.* New York: Guilford Press.

Moore, R., & Garland, A. (2003). *Cognitive therapy for chronic and persistent depression.* New York: John Wiley & Sons, Inc.

Papageorgiou, C., & Wells, A. (2003). *Depressive rumination: Nature, theory and treatment.* New York: John Wiley & Sons, Inc.

Persons, J. B., Davidson, J., & Tomkins, M. A. (2001). *Essential components of cognitive-behavioral therapy for depression.* Washington, D.C.: American Psychological Association.

Segal, Z. V., Williams, J. Mark G., & Teasdale, J. D. (2002). *Mindfulness-based cognitive therapy for depression: A new approach to preventing relapse.* New York: Guilford Press.

EATING DISORDERS

Cooper, M., Todd, G., & Wells, A. (2000). *Bulimia nervosa: A cognitive therapy programme for clients.* Philadelphia: Jessica Kingsley Publishers.

Cooper, Z., Fairburn, C. G., & Hawker, D. M. (2004). *Cognitive-behavioral treatment of obesity: A clinician's guide.* New York: Guilford Press.

Fairburn, C., & Brownell, K. (Eds.). (2002). *Eating disorders and obesity: A comprehensive handbook* (2nd ed.). New York: Guilford Press.

Fairburn, C., & Wilson, G. (Eds.). (1996). *Binge eating: Nature, assessment, and treatment.* New York: Guilford Press.

Garner, D. M., & Garfinkle, P. (Eds.). (1997). Handbook of treatment for eating disorders (2nd ed.). New York: Guilford Press.

Garner, D. M., Vitousek, K. M., & Pike, K. M. (1997). Cognitive-behavioral therapy for anorexia nervosa. In Garner, D. M. & Garfinkel, P. E. (Eds.), *Handbook of psychotherapy for anorexia nervosa and bulimia*. (pp. 94–144). New York: Guilford Press.

GROUP THERAPY

Free, M. E. (2000). *Cognitive therapy in groups: Guidelines and resources for practice.* New York: John Wiley & Sons, Inc.

White, J., & Freeman, A. (2000). *Cognitive-behavioral group therapy for specific problems and populations.* Washington, D.C.: American Psychological Association.

LEARNING AND INTELLECTUAL DISABILITIES

Kroese B., Dagnan, D., Loumidis, K., et al. (Eds.). (1977). *Cognitive-behaviour therapy for people with learning disabilities.* London: Routledge.

Radnitz, C. (Ed.). (2000). *Cognitive-behavioral therapy for persons with disabilities.* London: Jacob Aronson.

Nezu, C. M., Nezu, A. M., & Gill-Weiss, M. J. (1992). *Psychopathology in persons with mental retardation: Clinical guidelines for assessment and treatment.* Champaign, IL: Research Press.

MARRIAGE AND FAMILY PROBLEMS

Baucom, D. H., & Bozicas, G. D. (1990). *Cognitive behavioral marital therapy.* New York: Brunner/Mazel.

Dattilio, F. M. (1998). *Case studies in couple and family therapy: Systemic and cognitive perspectives.* New York: Guilford Press.

Dattilio, F. M., & Padesky, C. A. (1990). *Cognitive therapy with couples.* Sarasota: Professional Resources Exchange, Inc.

Epstein, N. B., & Baucom, D. H. (2002). *Enhanced cognitive-behavioral therapy for couples: A contextual approach.* Washington, D.C.: American Psychological Association.

Epstein, N. E., Schlesinger, S. E., & Dryden, W. (Eds.). (1988). *Cognitive-behavioral therapy with families.* New York: Brunner/Mazel.

MEDICAL PROBLEMS

Crawford, I., & Fishman, B. (Eds.). (1996). *Psychosocial interventions for HIV disease: A stage-focused and culture specific approach (cognitive behavioral therapy).* Jason Aronson Publishing.

Henry, J. L., & Wilson, P. H. (2000). *Psychological management of chronic tinnitus: A cognitive-behavioral approach.* Pearson Allyn & Bacon.

Moorey, S., & Greer, S. (2002). *Cognitive behaviour therapy for people with cancer.* Oxford, England: Oxford University Press.

Segal, Z. V., Toner, B. B., Shelagh, D. E., & Myran, D. (1999). *Cognitive-behavioral treatment of irritable bowel syndrome: The brain–gut connection.* New York: Guilford Press.

White, C. A. (2001). *Cognitive behaviour therapy for chronic medical problems.* Chichester, England: John Wiley & Sons, Inc.

Winterowd, C., Beck, A., & Gruener, D. (2003). *Cognitive therapy with chronic pain patients.* New York: Springer Publishing Company.

OLDER ADULTS

Laidlaw, K., Thompson, L. W., Dick-Siskin, L., & Gallagher-Thompson, D. (2003). *Cognitive behaviour therapy with older people.* Chicester, England: John Wiley & Sons, Inc.

Yost, E. B., Beutler, L. E., Corbishley, M. A., & Allender, J. R. (1987). *Group cognitive therapy: A treatment approach for depressed older adults.* New York: Pergamon Press.

PAIN

Thorn, B. E. (2004). *Cognitive therapy for chronic pain: A step-by-step guide.* New York: Guilford Press.

Winderowd, C., Beck, A. T., & Gruener, D. (2003). *Cognitive therapy with chronic pain patients.* New York: Springer Publishing Co.

PERSONALITY DISORDERS

Beck, A. T., Freeman, A., Davis, D. D., & Associates. (2003). *Cognitive therapy of personality disorders* (2nd ed.). New York: Guilford Press.

Layden, M. A., Newman, C. F., Freeman, A., & Morse, S. B. (1993). *Cognitive therapy of borderline personality disorder.* Boston, MA: Allyn & Bacon.

Linehan, M. (1993). *Cognitive-behavioral treatment of borderline personality disorder.* New York: Guilford Press.

Rasmusses, P. (2005). *Personality-guided cognitive-behavioral therapy.* Washington, D.C.: American Psychological Association.

Smucker, M. R., & Dancu, C. V. (1999). *Cognitive behavioral treatment of adult survivors of childhood trauma: Imagery rescripting and reprocessing.* Jason Aronson Publishing.

Sperry, L. (1999). *Cognitive behavior therapy of DSM-IV personality disorders.* New York: Brunner-Routledge.

Young, J., Klosko, J., & Weishaar, M. E. (2003). *Schema therapy: A practitioner's guide.* New York: Guilford Press.

RESISTANCE

Leahy, R. L. (2001). *Overcoming resistance in cognitive therapy.* New York: Guilford Press.

Leahy, R. L. (2003). *Roadblocks in cognitive-behavioral therapy: Transforming challenges into opportunities for change.* New York: Guilford Press.

SCHIZOPHRENIA

Chadwick, P., Birchwood, M., & Trower, P. (1996). *Cognitive therapy of delusions, voices, and paranoia.* New York: John Wiley & Sons, Inc.

Fowler, D., Garety, P., & Kuipers, E. (1995). *Cognitive behavior therapy for psychosis: Theory and practice.* New York: John Wiley & Sons, Inc.

French, P., & Morrison, A. (2004). *Early detection and cognitive therapy for people at high risk for psychosis: A treatment approach.* New York: John Wiley & Sons, Inc.

Haddock, G., & Slade, P. D. (Eds.). (1996). *Cognitive behavioral interventions with psychotic disorders.* New York: Routledge.

Kingdon, D. G., & Turkington, D. (1994). *Cognitive-behavioral therapy of schizophrenia.* Mahwah, NJ: Lawrence Erlbaum Associates.

Kingdon, D., & Turkington, D. (Eds.). (2002). *A case study guide to cognitive behavioural therapy of psychosis.* New York: John Wiley & Sons, Inc.

Kingdon, D., & Turkington, D. (2005). *Cognitive therapy of schizophrenia.* New York: Guilford Press.

Marco, M. C. G., Perris, C., & Brenner, B. (Eds.). (2002). *Cognitive therapy with schizophrenic patients: The evolution of a new treatment approach.* Hogrefe & Huber Publications.

Morrison, A. (2002). *A casebook of cognitive therapy for psychosis.* New York: Brunner-Routledge.

Morrison, A. P. (2004). *Cognitive therapy for psychosis: A formulation-based approach.* New York: Brunner-Routledge.

Nelson, H. (1997). *Cognitive behavioral therapy with schizophrenia.* Chetenham, England: Stanley Thornes Ltd.

Perris, C., McGorry, P., & Jackson, H. (Eds.). (2005). *The recognition and management of early psychosis: A preventive approach.* Cambridge, England: Cambridge University Press.

SUBSTANCE ABUSE

Beck, A. T., Wright, F. D., Newman, C. F., & Liese, B. S. (1993). *Cognitive therapy of substance abuse.* New York: Guilford Press.

Najavits, L. M. (2001). *Seeking safety: A treatment manual for PTSD and substance abuse.* New York: Guilford Press.

Thase, M. (1997). Cognitive-behavioral therapy for substance abuse disorders. In Dickstein, L. J., Riba, M. B., & Oldham, J. M. (Eds.), *Review of psychiatry,* Vol. 16, (pp. I-45–I-72). Washington, D.C.: American Psychiatric Press.

MISCELLANEOUS

Bedrosian, R. C., & Bozicas, G. (1994). *Treating family of origin problems: A cognitive approach.* New York: Guilford Press.

Freeman, A., & Dattilio, F. M. (Eds.). (2000). Cognitive-behavioral strategies in crisis intervention (2nd ed.). New York: Guilford Press.

Dattilio, F. M., & Freeman, A. (Eds.). (2000). *Cognitive-behavioral strategies in crisis intervention* (2nd ed.). New York: Guilford Press.

Kroese, B. S., Dagnan, D., & Loumides, K. (Eds.). (1997). *Cognitive behaviour therapy for people with learning disabilities.* London: Routledge.

Martell, C. R., Safran, S. A., & Prince, S. E. (2003). *Cognitive-behavioral therapies with lesbian, gay, and bisexual clients.* New York: Guilford Press.

Radnitz, C. L. (Ed.). (2000). *Cognitive behavioral therapy for persons with disabilities.* Jason Aronson Publishing.

Safran, J. D., & Segal, Z. V. (1996). *Interpersonal process in cognitive therapy.* Jason Aronson Publishing.

Wills, F., & Sanders, D. (1997). *Cognitive therapy: Transforming the image.* London: Sage Publications.

Wright, J. H., Thase, M. E., Beck, A. T., & Ludgate, J. W. (1993). *Cognitive therapy with inpatients: Developing a cognitive milieu.* New York: Guilford Press.

CLINICAL APPLICATIONS: BOOKS COVERING MULTIPLE DISORDERS, PROBLEMS, OR POPULATIONS

Beck, A.T. (1976). *Cognitive therapy and the emotional disorders.* New York: International Universities Press.

Blackburn, I. M., Twaddle, V., & Associates. (1996). *Cognitive therapy in action. A practitioner's casebook.* London: Souvenier Press (Educational & Academic), Ltd.

Bennett-Levy, J., Butler, G., Fennell, M., Hackmann, A., Mueller, M. & Westbrook, D. (Eds.). (2004). *Oxford guide to behavioural experiments in cognitive therapy.* Oxford, England: Oxford University Press.

Caballo, V. E. (Ed.). (1998). *International handbook of cognitive and behavioural treatments for psychological disorders.* Oxford, England: Pergamon/Elsevier Science.

Clark, D. M., & Fairburn, C. G. (Eds.). (1997). *Science and practice of cognitive behavior therapy.* New York: Oxford University Press.

Freeman, A. (2005). *Encyclopedia of cognitive behavior therapy.* New York: Plenum Press.

Freeman, A., & Dattilio, F. M. (1992). *Comprehensive casebook of cognitive therapy.* New York: Plenum Press.

Freeman, A., Pretzer, J., Fleming, B., & Simon, K. M. (1990). *Clinical applications of cognitive therapy.* New York: Plenum Press.

Freeman, A., Simon, K. M., Beutler, L., & Arkowitz, H. (Eds.). (1989). *Comprehensive handbook of cognitive therapy.* New York: Plenum Publishers.

Granvold, D. K. (Ed.). (1998). *Cognitive and behavioral treatment: Methods and applications.* Wadsworth Publishing.

Kuehlwein, K. T., & Rosen, H. (Eds.). (1993). *Cognitive therapies in action: Evolving innovative practice.* San Francisco: Jossey-Bass.

Leahy, R. (1996). *Cognitive therapy: Basic principles and applications.* Northvale, NJ: Jason Aronson Inc.

Leahy, R. (Ed.). (1997). *Practicing cognitive therapy: A guide to interventions.* Northvale, NJ: Jason Aronson Inc.

Leahy, R. (Ed.). (2004). *Contemporary cognitive therapy.* New York: Guilford Press.

Leahy, R. L., & Dowd, T. E. (Eds.). (2002). *Clinical advances in cognitive psychotherapy: Theory and application.* New York: Springer Publishing Company.

Leahy, R. L., & Holland, S. J. (2000). *Treatment plans and interventions for depression and anxiety disorders.* New York: Guilford Press.

Lyddon, W. J., & Jones, J. V. (Eds.). (2001). *Empirically supported cognitive therapies: Current and future applications.* New York: Springer Publishing.

Reinecke, M., & Clark, D. (Eds.). (2003). *Cognitive therapy across the lifespan: Evidence and practice.* Cambridge, England: Cambridge University Press.

Salkovskis, P. M. (Ed.). (1996). *Frontiers of cognitive therapy.* New York: Guilford Press.

Salkovskis, P. M. (Ed.). (1996). *Trends in cognitive therapy and behavioural therapies.* New York: John Wiley & Sons, Inc.

Scott, J., Williams, M. G., & Beck, A. T. (Eds.). (1989). *Cognitive therapy in clinical practice.* New York: Routledge.

Simos, G. (Ed.). (2002). *Cognitive behaviour therapy: A guide for the practicing clinician.* New York: Brunner-Routledge.

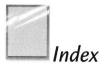
Index

Page numbers followed by *f* indicate figure.